FIFTH EDITION

FACILITATOR GUIDE FOR
JOHNS HOPKINS EVIDENCE-BASED PRACTICE

FOR NURSES AND HEALTHCARE PROFESSIONALS

Model & Guidelines

Kim Bissett, PhD, MBA, RN
Judith Ascenzi, DNP, RN
Madeleine Whalen, MSN/MPH, RN, CEN, NPD-BC

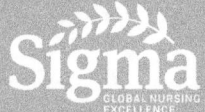

Copyright © 2025 by Sigma Theta Tau International Honor Society of Nursing

All rights reserved. This book is protected by copyright. No part of it may be reproduced, stored in a retrieval system, or transmitted in any form or by any means, electronic, mechanical, photocopying, recording, or otherwise, without written permission from the publisher. Any trademarks, service marks, design rights, or similar rights that are mentioned, used, or cited in this book are the property of their respective owners. Their use here does not imply that you may use them for a similar or any other purpose.

This book is not intended to be a substitute for the medical advice of a licensed medical professional. The author and publisher have made every effort to ensure the accuracy of the information contained within at the time of its publication and shall have no liability or responsibility to any person or entity regarding any loss or damage incurred, or alleged to have incurred, directly or indirectly, by the information contained in this book. The author and publisher make no warranties, express or implied, with respect to its content, and no warranties may be created or extended by sales representatives or written sales materials. The author and publisher have no responsibility for the consistency or accuracy of URLs and content of third-party websites referenced in this book.

Sigma Theta Tau International Honor Society of Nursing (Sigma) is a nonprofit organization whose mission is developing nurse leaders anywhere to improve healthcare everywhere. Founded in 1922, Sigma has more than 80,000 active members in over 100 countries and territories. Members include practicing nurses, instructors, researchers, policymakers, entrepreneurs, and others. Sigma's 600 chapters are located at more than 700 institutions of higher education throughout Armenia, Australia, Botswana, Brazil, Canada, Chile, Colombia, Croatia, England, Eswatini, Finland, Ghana, Hong Kong, Ireland, Israel, Italy, Jamaica, Japan, Jordan, Kenya, Lebanon, Malawi, Mexico, the Netherlands, Nigeria, Pakistan, Philippines, Portugal, Puerto Rico, Saudi Arabia, Scotland, Singapore, South Africa, South Korea, Spain, Sweden, Taiwan, Tanzania, Thailand, the United States, and Wales. Learn more at www.sigmanursing.org.

Sigma Theta Tau International
550 West North Street
Indianapolis, IN, USA 46202

To request a review copy for course adoption, order additional books, buy in bulk, or purchase for corporate use, contact Sigma Marketplace at 888.654.4968 (US/Canada toll-free), +1.317.687.2256 (International), or solutions@sigmamarketplace.org.

To request author information, or for speaker or other media requests, contact Sigma Marketing at 888.634.7575 (US/Canada toll-free) or +1.317.634.8171 (International).

ISBN: 9781646481361
EPUB ISBN: 9781646481378

Publisher: Dustin Sullivan
Acquisitions Editor: Emily Hatch
Development Editor: Jillmarie Leeper Sycamore
Cover Designer: Rebecca Batchelor
Interior Design/Page Layout: Rebecca Batchelor

Managing Editor: Carla Hall
Publications Specialist: Todd Lothery
Project Editor: Todd Lothery
Copy Editor: Todd Lothery
Proofreader: Todd Lothery

DEDICATION

This book is dedicated to nurses and healthcare professionals everywhere—in whatever setting they practice—who are committed to excellence in patient care based on the best available evidence.

ABOUT THE AUTHORS

Kim Bissett, PhD, MBA, RN, is a nurse educator and Director of EBP at the Institute for Johns Hopkins Nursing. She has been involved with the Johns Hopkins Evidence-Based Practice (JHEBP) model for many years including as an EBP Fellow, a hospital-based EBP Coordinator, and a workshop facilitator. She has extensive experience in EBP education, presenting and consulting on evidence-based nursing practice nationally and internationally. Bissett assisted with developing and publishing previous editions of the *Johns Hopkins Nursing Evidence-Based Practice: Model and Guidelines.* She also teaches part time in the Johns Hopkins University School of Nursing's Doctor of Nursing Practice Program. Her research interests include self-compassion and fostering nurse well-being.

Judith Ascenzi, DNP, RN, is the Director of Pediatric Nursing Programs for Education, Informatics, and Research at the Johns Hopkins Children's Center. She also teaches part time in the Johns Hopkins University School of Nursing's Doctorate of Nursing Practice Program. Ascenzi has presented and consulted nationally on the topic of evidence-based practice. She has served as expert facilitator on many evidence-based practice projects in her pediatric practice setting as well as with her adult colleagues at the Johns Hopkins Hospital. Ascenzi acts as a project advisor and organizational mentor for many doctoral students utilizing the JHEBP model as the foundational model for their projects.

Madeleine Whalen, MSN/MPH, RN, CEN, NPD-BC, is the Evidence-Based Practice Program Coordinator for the Johns Hopkins Health System. In this role she educates and supports frontline nurses in completing robust and actionable EBP projects rooted in bedside experience. She began her nursing career in the emergency department while earning her master's degrees in nursing and public health. She is a Joanna Briggs Institute Scientific Writer and a member of the *Journal of Emergency Nursing* editorial board. She continues to work clinically part-time as well as serves as adjunct faculty at the Johns Hopkins School of Nursing and the Johns Hopkins Medicine Center for Global Emergency Care. Her professional interests include global health, evidence synthesis, and empowering nurses to advance the profession and science of nursing through inquiry.

CONTRIBUTING AUTHORS

Brenda Douglass, DNP, APRN, FNP-C, CDCES, CNE, CTTS, is a Family Nurse Practitioner, Assistant Professor, and Associate Director of the DNP-AP Program - Project Focus at the Johns Hopkins University School of Nursing. She brings a wealth of experience and leadership, integrating academic, clinical, research, and leadership roles throughout her career. A recognized leader in nursing education, she provides program oversight of DNP projects, project core courses, and practicum experiences, ensuring alignment with accreditation standards, competency-based education, and evidence-based practice. Douglass is actively involved in advancing DNP education through initiatives focused on enhancing project and practicum experiences, integrating competency-based education, and strengthening academic-practice partnerships. Douglass serves on national and university committees focused on nursing education, leadership, and policy and is a dedicated mentor and advisor committed to developing future nurse leaders and educators who are prepared to drive healthcare transformation through evidence-based practice and quality improvement initiatives.

Lisa Grubb, DNP, MSN, BSN, RN, CWCN, CPHQ, C/DONA, is an Assistant Professor at the Johns Hopkins University School of Nursing, where she coordinates and teaches in the DNP/AP project courses. She uses the Johns Hopkins Evidence-Based Practice model as a foundation for all DNP project courses. Before her current role, she was the Senior Director of Quality and Patient Safety at the Johns Hopkins Howard County Medical Center, where she focused on using evidence-based practices to improve patient outcomes, including reducing length of stay, decreasing readmissions, and enhancing patient satisfaction and value-based care. Additionally, she has collaborated with the Institute for Johns Hopkins Nursing and the Johns Hopkins Nursing Administration to support nurses in evidence-based practice, knowledge translation, and quality improvement research projects. Grubb has a strong interest in promoting EBP in both clinical settings and academic environments.

Alexandra Johnson, MPH, MSN, RN, is a Program Coordinator for the Department of Nursing at the Johns Hopkins Hospital. In this role, she conducts and guides nursing research, evidence-based practice, and quality improvement work. Originally from Chicago, Illinois, Alexandra relocated to Maryland in 2018 to join the Johns Hopkins Hospital as a nurse in the neonatal intensive care unit, where she continues to work clinically part-time. Alexandra is also adjunct faculty at the Johns Hopkins University School of Nursing.

Hayley D. Mark, PhD, MPH, RN, FAAN, is a Professor in the Towson University Department of Nursing. She previously served as the Chair of the TU Department of Nursing and the Director of the Baccalaureate Program at Johns Hopkins University School of Nursing. Mark is nationally recognized for her scholarship on sexual health and nursing education. She has been funded by the National Institutes of Health and the Centers for Disease Control and Prevention and is widely published on topics related to serological testing for the herpes simplex virus, HPV testing, and cervical cancer screening. Mark is a Fellow in the American Academic of Nursing.

Hyunjeong Park, PhD, MPH, MSN, RN, is an Associate Professor and the Chair of the Department of Nursing at Towson University. With extensive expertise in the fields of cultural diversity, health-related behaviors, and immigrant health management, Park has made significant contributions to understanding the intersection of culture and healthcare. Park has also played a pivotal role in the development of instrument measurement studies that have been widely adopted across a range of academic disciplines and healthcare contexts. Park has a strong record of collaboration with global scholars, engaging in cross-cultural research and co-authoring numerous publications. She is dedicated to advancing knowledge in her field and promoting health equity through evidence-based practices.

TABLE OF CONTENTS

About the Authors iv
Contributing Authors v
Introduction to the Facilitator Guide vii
Chapter Summaries viii

Part 1 Undergraduate Education 1

Part 2 Graduate Education 7
    Master's Education Teaching Guide 7
    Doctoral Education Teaching Guide 12

Part 3 Professional Development for Healthcare Organizations 25

Part 4 Workbook Learning Activities and Answer Key 39

Part 5 Sample DNP Scholarly Project Curriculum Outline 101

    References 137

INTRODUCTION TO THE FACILITATOR GUIDE

Johns Hopkins Evidence-Based Practice for Nurses and Healthcare Professionals: Model & Guidelines, 5th Edition, reaffirms the original mission of the Johns Hopkins Evidence-Based Practice (JHEBP) model to support patient safety, professional development, and the education of healthcare students. Many evidence-based practice (EBP) books are in print today, but what makes this book valuable is its applicability for use in the classroom and its practical approach for the practice setting. The detailed guidelines and specific tools that accompany each step in the process promote success.

This facilitator guide is intended for use by university faculty and nurses and healthcare clinicians facilitating professional development in healthcare organizations. The main book is used as a text for undergraduate, graduate, and doctoral courses to help students achieve the knowledge, skills, and abilities necessary to learn the essentials of their educational programs. The JHEBP model is also used in the practice environment to guide clinical inquiry and enhance practice decision-making. The model and tools have high utility in both environments.

Parts 1 and 2 of this guide offer details about incorporating EBP content throughout baccalaureate, master's, and doctoral curricula. They include suggestions for teaching EBP and leveling the content depending on student knowledge and previous experience with EBP, as well as examples of course objectives, assignments, and grading rubrics. Part 3 provides a discussion and practical examples for infusing EBP throughout an organization as part of a professional development program. Part 4 contains the learning activities, with an answer key, from the workbook for *Johns Hopkins Evidence-Based Practice for Nurses and Healthcare Professionals: Model & Guidelines,* 5th Edition. Part 5 presents a detailed sample DNP scholarly project curriculum outline. We hope that you find this facilitator guide a useful and exciting addition to the textbook. What follows are the key points for each chapter of the textbook, which are also listed at the beginning of each chapter in the book.

CHAPTER SUMMARIES

CHAPTER 1
EVIDENCE-BASED PRACTICE: PAST, PRESENT, AND FUTURE

Key Points
- Evidence-based practice (EBP) helps clinicians keep up with emerging evidence, practices, and technologies.
- The Johns Hopkins Evidence-Based Practice (JHEBP) Model for Nursing and Healthcare Professionals provides a structured and systematic way for clinicians to effectively use current scientific and experiential evidence to determine best practices and provide safe, high-quality care.
- Numerous healthcare organizations encourage the use and prioritization of EBP.
- EBP can be used during resource-limited times such as with the COVID-19 pandemic. Clinicians may need to think creatively and expand their skill sets.
- Artificial intelligence (AI) can potentially enhance the EBP process by speeding up the process or replacing many of the human tasks. In the future, AI may complete entire EBP projects in seconds.
- EBP teams can address health equity locally by considering diversity, equity, and inclusion from the start of the EBP project.

CHAPTER 2
THE JOHNS HOPKINS EVIDENCE-BASED PRACTICE (JHEBP) MODEL FOR NURSES AND HEALTHCARE PROFESSIONALS (HCPs) PROCESS OVERVIEW

Key Points
This chapter summarizes all the steps in the JHEBP model. The JHEBP Project Steps and Overview (Appendix A) mirrors this overview.

- QI, research, and EBP are the three forms of inquiry common to healthcare.
- The JHEBP model is built on the concepts of inquiry, practice, and learning.
- Critical thinking and clinical reasoning are essential components of the model.
- The EBP process can be influenced by both internal and external factors.
- The JHEBP model uses the PET process: Practice Question, Evidence, and Translation.
- The JHEBP model consists of 16 steps with associated tools to guide the EBP process.

CHAPTER 3
PRACTICE QUESTION PHASE: THE PROBLEM

Key Points

The practice question phase contains three steps. This chapter reviews the first and second steps. The JHEBP Question Development Tool (Appendix B) facilitates this phase.

- Failing to fully describe and define the problem can lead to ineffective solutions.
- Teams should avoid starting with a solution in mind, focusing on the symptoms of the problem, and jumping on the first problem identified.
- Spending time exploring the problem with techniques such as a root cause analysis will help identify the true problem.
- Inaccurate or poorly defined problem statements may lead to wasted time, resources, and potential dead ends in the EBP process.

CHAPTER 4
PRACTICE QUESTION PHASE: THE EBP QUESTION

Key Points

The practice question phase contains three steps. This chapter covers the final step. The JHEBP Question Development Tool (Appendix B) facilitates this step.

- In many instances, PICO—Patient/Population/Problem, Intervention, Comparison, and Outcome—has become synonymous with the EBP question, with teams using "PICO question" and "EBP question" interchangeably. However, PICO guides searches. It doesn't support question development as well.
- Searchable questions are concise and focused, possibly limited to two to three main ideas.
- Broad (formerly background questions) EBP questions cast a wide net and provide a good starting point.
- Intervention (formerly foreground) EBP questions provide more precise knowledge to drive decision-making.
- Before embarking on a full EBP project, teams should examine the project's potential alignment with organizational priorities, impact on outcomes, and ability to be implemented in the current climate.

CHAPTER 5
THE INTERPROFESSIONAL TEAM

Key Points

- It is critical to build an interprofessional team to collaborate with embarking on an EBP project.
- When building core EBP team members and selecting the team leader, consider their expertise, influence, character traits, behavior traits, and team dynamics.

- Consider impacted groups that may influence or be influenced by the EBP project. Impacted groups can include patients, families, managers, and policymakers.
- Impacted groups can broaden the team's perspective, enhance the project's impact, and make the audience feel inclusive and considerate of all perspectives.
- Recognizing and appreciating contributions within the team enhances belonging and commitment to the project.
- Successful teams tend to have a clear vision and direction.

CHAPTER 6
EVIDENCE PHASE: INTRODUCTION TO EVIDENCE

Key Points
The evidence phase contains seven steps. This chapter gives an overview of the evidence that will be gathered and appraised in Steps 4, 5, and 6. Information in this chapter will assist the EBP team in completing the JHEBP Searching and Screening Tool (Appendix C) and the Pre-appraised Evidence Appraisal Tool, Single Study Evidence Appraisal Tool, and Anecdotal Evidence Appraisal Tool (Appendices E1, E2, and E3, respectively).

- The JHEBP model has updated its approach to evidence appraisal.
- Pre-appraised evidence—such as clinical practice guidelines (CPGs), literature reviews with a systematic approach (LRSAs), and evidence summaries—can provide independent support for decision-making if they are suitable to the EBP question and of sufficient quality.
- There are various types of LRSAs, but all must meet specific criteria to be considered "systematic."
- Single studies with formal study designs can provide strong or moderate support for decision-making if they are of sufficient quality.
- Studies may follow qualitative, quantitative, or mixed-methods approaches.
- Anecdotal evidence—such as expert opinions, book chapters, position statements, case reports, programmatic experiences, or literature reviews without a systematic approach—provides limited support for decision-making.

CHAPTER 7
EVIDENCE PHASE: THE EVIDENCE SEARCH AND SCREENING

Key Points
The evidence phase contains seven steps. This chapter covers the first two. The JHEBP Searching and Screening Tool (Appendix C) facilitates these steps.

- There are various types of literature searches an EBP team can conduct, yet all should follow a systematic process to promote efficiency and minimize bias.

- Best-evidence literature searches concentrate on gathering foundational information and pre-appraised evidence. Various databases specialize in providing this type of evidence.
- Exhaustive evidence literature searches attempt to gather all literature on a topic within pre-determined parameters. EBP teams design search strategies to conduct these searches.
- The EBP question guides the literature search. EBP teams will need to isolate the elements of their EBP question to create search concepts and build search strings.
- Additional tools to create search strings include truncation, Boolean operators, controlled vocabulary, exact phrasing, and title/abstract limiters.
- Literature screening is a systematic process to winnow down the results of an exhaustive search in an unbiased manner to only those that answer the EBP question and meet inclusion/exclusion criteria.
- Documenting the search and screening process is an important element to establish rigor and replicability.
- Various forms of bias can influence the trustworthiness of the results of a team's literature search. Bias should be recognized and minimized.

CHAPTER 8
EVIDENCE PHASE: APPRAISING THE EVIDENCE

Key Points

The evidence phase contains seven steps. This chapter discusses Step 6. The JHEBP Appraisal Tool Selection Algorithm (Appendix D), Pre-appraised Evidence Appraisal Tool (Appendix E1), Single Study Evidence Appraisal Tool (Appendix E2), Anecdotal Evidence Appraisal Tool (Appendix E3), and Evidence Terminology and Considerations Guide (Appendix F) facilitate these steps.

- The appraisal process consists of determining the level of support for decision-making evidence and assessing the quality of that evidence to ensure it is adequate.
- The specific action items of the process will vary depending on the type of evidence the team is appraising.
- Pre-appraised evidence requires a suitability assessment and a quality assessment.
- Single studies with a formal study design require an assessment of the design to determine the level of support for decision-making, followed by a quality assessment.
- Anecdotal evidence requires a quality assessment.

CHAPTER 9
EVIDENCE PHASE: SUMMARY, SYNTHESIS, AND BEST-EVIDENCE RECOMMENDATIONS

Key Points

The evidence phase contains seven steps. This chapter provides an overview of Steps 7–10. The JHEBP Best-Evidence Summary Tool (Appendix G1), Individual Evidence Summary Tool (Appendix G2), and Summary, Synthesis, & Best-Evidence Recommendations Tool (Appendix H) facilitate these steps.

- *Evidence summary* is the process of collating essential information from articles or reports into a central location. The EBP team uses a table with headers to provide pertinent data.
- Organizing or preparing the data from the evidence summary assists the team in conducting the next step of the process, evidence synthesis. This can be done with various visual and sorting tools.
- *Synthesis* is the process of creating greater meaning from the data provided by individual articles or reports.
- Synthesized evidence is used to generate best-evidence recommendations that answer the EBP question. Recommendations can be high, reasonable, reasonable-to-low, or low certainty.

CHAPTER 10
TRANSLATION PHASE: TRANSLATION

Key Points

The translation phase contains six steps. This chapter gives an overview of Steps 11–12 to develop practice setting-specific recommendations from the evidence synthesis. Information in this chapter will assist the EBP team in completing the Translation Tool (Appendix I).

- *Translation* is the process of adapting or customizing evidence findings into the specific content into which they will be implemented.
- The EBP team needs to follow these steps to ensure that effective translation of each piece of evidence occurs:
  - Consider the certainty of each best-evidence recommendation.
  - Identify the potential negative impact on patient or staff safety.
  - *Fit* is accomplished by evaluating both the end-user and organizational characteristics.
  - Assessing the practice environment's readiness to change is critical to determining the feasibility of evidence translation.
  - Impacted groups are essential when establishing acceptability of the evidence.
- Tools exist that the EBP team can use to help inform organizational decision-making related to translation. The EBP team should make organization-specific recommendations and record them to ensure that all are clear so that implementation may proceed.

CHAPTER 11
TRANSLATION PHASE: IMPLEMENTATION

Key Points

The translation phase contains six steps. This chapter provides an overview of the final steps (13–16) to implement any changes identified in Step 12. Information in this chapter will assist the EBP team in completing the JHEBP Implementation and Action Planning (A3) Tool (Appendix J).

- Selecting the correct project management tools is crucial for successful EBP implementation.
- The *A3 tool* is a project plan that consolidates the entire project implementation into one tool.
- A detailed project timeline can be incorporated into the project's A3.
- A *Gantt chart* is a high-level visual representation where a Work Breakdown Structure is more granular in identifying specific tasks and when they need to be completed.
- Identifying an implementation framework to help guide your project implementation can enhance the efficiency, effectiveness, and sustainability of your implementation.
- The *TRIP model* is an implementation framework that works well with the JHEBP model.
- A sustainability plan is imperative to ensure that project changes outlast the closure of the project.

CHAPTER 12
ONGOING CONSIDERATIONS: COMMUNICATION AND DISSEMINATION

Key Points

Dissemination can occur throughout the EBP project. Resources to facilitate the process include the Impacted Groups Analysis and Communication Resource and the EBP Reporting Guidelines provided in the additional resources online (Hopkins.org/resources).

- There are five components of an effective dissemination plan, including purpose, message, audience, timing, and method.
- *Internal dissemination* refers to sharing information with groups within a team's organization.
- Communication strategies should be tailored for unit-, departmental-, and organization-level groups. Executive summaries can be an effective communication strategy for executive leadership.

- *External dissemination* refers to sharing information outside a team's organization.
- Venues for external dissemination include conferences, peer-reviewed journals, and social media.
- Communication and dissemination are essential components of an EBP project. Not only are they mandates by healthcare associations, such as the American Nurses Association, but they are also essential for improving care for patients and advancing the science of healthcare.

CHAPTER 13
EXEMPLARS

Summary

This chapter presents six project exemplars using the 4th edition of *Johns Hopkins Evidence-Based Practice for Nurses and Healthcare Professionals: Model & Guidelines.* While these good examples of the JHEBP model do not include the new tools and terminology changes from the new edition, the overall process remains the same. Each exemplar:

- Highlights the use of the JHEBP model in real-world EBP projects
- Provides an example of one way to document an EBP project

APPENDICES

Appendices include project planning guides, flowcharts, decision supports, specific directions, and support for step-by-step implementation of the JHEBP model:

- Appendix A: EBP Project Steps and Overview
- Appendix B: Question Development Tool
- Appendix C: Searching and Screening Tool
- Appendix D: Appraisal Tool Selection Algorithm
- Appendix E1: Pre-appraised Evidence Appraisal Tool
- Appendix E2: Single Study Evidence Appraisal Tool
- Appendix E3: Anecdotal Evidence Appraisal Tool
- Appendix F: Evidence Terminology and Considerations Guide
- Appendix G1: Best-Evidence Summary Tool
- Appendix G2: Individual Evidence Summary Tool
- Appendix H: Summary, Synthesis, & Best-Evidence Recommendations Tool
- Appendix I: Translation Tool
- Appendix J: Implementation and Action Planning (A3) Tool

PART I
UNDERGRADUATE EDUCATION

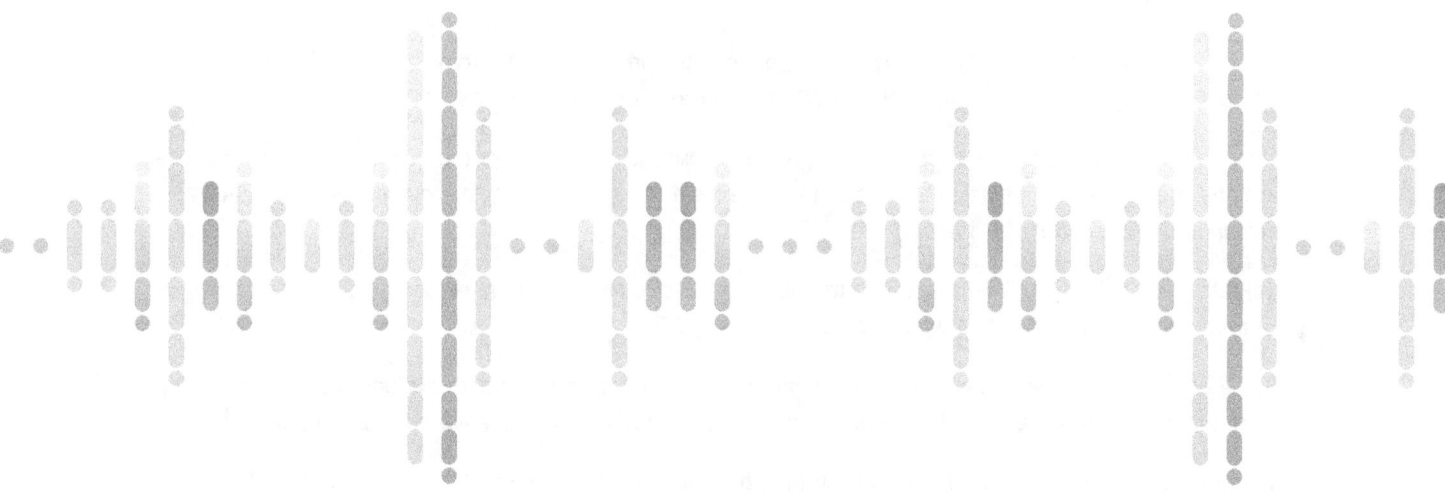

BACCALAUREATE EDUCATION TEACHING GUIDE

Evidence-based practice (EBP) is one of the American Association of Colleges of Nursing's (AACN) *Essentials of Baccalaureate Education for Professional Nursing Practice* because professional nursing practice is grounded in the translation of current evidence into one's practice (AACN, 2008). EBP, an organizing structure to examine nursing practice, should be integrated into all aspects of undergraduate nursing education. In undergraduate-level nursing programs, EBP is often introduced in a first-semester course to lay a strong foundation for how it applies to the role of a professional nurse. It may then be threaded throughout the curriculum in didactic and clinical courses. EBP and research skills—including research methodology, the EBP process, and its application to a clinical question—may be taught in the second semester. As students expand their clinical skills in the third semester, they may continue to examine evidence for nursing practice at their clinical sites. In some programs in the fourth semester, students must take a seminar course that involves completing an EBP project. Nursing students often find it difficult to understand the concept of EBP and are challenged to apply it in a meaningful way because of their inexperience in practice. The usefulness of the book *Johns Hopkins Evidence-Based Practice for Nurses and Healthcare Professionals: Model & Guidelines,* 5th Edition, is underscored by its simplicity and language, free of research jargon. Students may use the book as a required textbook along with a foundational nursing research text. As each topic is discussed, readings are selected to supplement the topic.

Research at the baccalaureate level is often offered as a three-credit course. Figure 1.1 provides an example of course objectives with associated program outcomes and the AACN *Essentials*. This course aims to introduce students to the scientific process, emphasizing its application in nursing. The steps of the research process may be presented along with research questions, major research designs (including experimental and quasi-experimental studies), and descriptive and qualitative designs.

SAMPLE BACCALAUREATE RESEARCH FOR EBP COURSE OBJECTIVES

After the course, the student will:

1. Distinguish differences among EBP, quality improvement, and nursing research in the profession of nursing. *(Associated program outcomes 4, 5; AACN Baccalaureate Essentials III)*

2. Compare and contrast major methods of nursing research. *(Associated program outcomes 4, 5; AACN Baccalaureate Essentials III)*

3. Apply an EBP model to identify and critically appraise the current literature for a specific clinical question. *(Associated program outcomes 4, 5, 9; AACN Baccalaureate Essentials III, VII)*

4. Apply knowledge of research ethics and basic research principles to improve the quality and safety of patient care and protect research participants across the life span. *(Associated program outcomes 7, 11; AACN Baccalaureate Essentials III, VIII, IX)*

5. Evaluate the reliability and validity of the measurement instruments used in a research study. *(Associated program outcome 6; AACN Baccalaureate Essentials III, IV)*

6. Utilize an understanding of basic statistical analysis, including descriptive and inferential statistics, to appraise the relevance of study results. *(Associated program outcome 6; AACN Baccalaureate Essentials III, IV)*

7. Communicate and disseminate findings from the application of the evidence-based process model to improve the quality and safety of care for diverse populations. *(Associated program outcomes 8, 10; AACN Baccalaureate Essentials III, VI, VIII)*

FIGURE 1.1 Sample baccalaureate research for EBP course objectives *(H. Park, personal communication, Nov. 3, 2024).*

The course emphasizes developing an understanding of the logical process of research, the importance of carrying out studies of nursing interest with scientific rigor, and how to critically read and incorporate research into practice.

For example, students may complete assigned readings on threats to internal validity and a research article. They can then spend class time discussing the threats and an overview of all threats provided as a summary of the class content. The application of content to research articles engages students. Students can use the same article discussed with the threats to highlight information recorded on the Johns Hopkins Evidence-Based Practice (JHEBP) Single Study Evidence Appraisal Tool (Appendix E2).

Students in some programs use the JHEBP tools during class as interactive exercises. For example, during the discussion of the purpose of research, students apply the section on developing an answerable EBP question using the Question Development Tool (Appendix B) on pages 212–213 of the book to identify a clinical concern. Students may use the JHEBP appraisal tools when critiquing studies for in-class exercises and for assignments.

Conducting an individual or group EBP project as a final learning activity in an undergraduate research course can help students develop skills that they will apply in clinical practice after graduation. One way to involve nursing students with an actual clinical issue is to have them work with registered nurses from affiliated healthcare organizations to generate clinical questions of concern. Faculty often find organizations' EBP committee chairs helpful in establishing this collaboration. Figure 1.2 includes EBP topics identified by affiliating hospitals. Students participate in an EBP project on a patient care unit and may cite their contribution in their portfolio. An overview of an EBP project that could be added to the course syllabus is included in Figure 1.3 with the grading rubric (Figure 1.4). Students often report that the actual EBP project is fun, and they appreciate the application of these principles to practice.

EBP QUESTIONS FROM AFFILIATING HEALTHCARE ORGANIZATIONS

- What is the best practice for utilizing computerized information systems (CPIs) to improve handoff communication involving high-risk medications when transferring patients?
- What is the most reliable and valid sedation assessment tool for pediatric ICU patients?
- What is the patient's/family's perception of healthcare workers' professional image/dress?
- What is the smallest size peripheral IV catheter that can be used in an adult for blood transfusion and prevention of hemolysis to the cells?
- What interventions have been implemented to manage disruptive behavior between and among professionals in the workplace?
- What are the best strategies to decrease errors in pathology specimen labeling?
- Does double-check verification of medication prior to administration decrease medication errors?
- What are the best chest pain stratification tools/guidelines for use at triage?
- What is the best practice for a feeding model that supports the infant's neurological development and is easily translatable to staff and parents?
- What is the best practice to improve international venous thromboembolism (I-VTE-1) compliance?
- What are the safe interventions in preventing falls in the ambulatory setting compared to current practice?
- How long can an asymptomatic peripheral intravenous access remain in place prior to site rotation among adult inpatients?

FIGURE 1.2 EBP questions from affiliating healthcare organizations.

GUIDELINES FOR GROUP EBP PROJECT

Purpose:

The purpose of the EBP project is to have the student demonstrate skills in applying research to practice. This is a group exercise. The PICO and all tools are available on the course website.

Procedures:

Students will work in teams of three to six. Each group will:

1. Identify a topic of interest using the PICO form. Topics may be clinical, management, or educational nursing practices.

2. Conduct a literature search on the chosen topic and select appropriate articles for critique. Include at least eight articles of evidence. Critique each article using the JHEBP tools. Include copies of the articles in the final report.

3. Complete the Individual Evidence Summary Tool (Appendix G2) that includes limitations, degree of decision-making support, and quality of evidence.

4. Complete the Summary, Synthesis, & Best-Evidence Recommendations Tool (Appendix H) that includes practice recommendations.

5. Evaluate each member's contribution to the group project, including your own.

The evidence report should be organized in a narrative report in the following way:

a. Abstract

b. Introduction (overview of clinical problem area)

c. Purpose
   - Relevance to nursing
   - Significance of project

d. Methodology
   - Description of literature review
   - Types and level of evidence found
   - Volume of research in the area

e. Brief results

f. Conclusion and implications for nursing (practice recommendation)

g. Reference list in APA format

h. Appendices:
   1. Individual Evidence Summary Tool
   2. Summary, Synthesis, & Best-Evidence Recommendations Tool
   3. Copy of each piece of evidence reviewed, with best-evidence recommendations for each article
   4. Peer reviews in individual, sealed envelopes

FIGURE 1.3 Guidelines for group EBP project.

GRADING RUBRIC FOR BACCALAUREATE-LEVEL EBP PROJECT	POSSIBLE POINTS

Executive summary
    Introduction
    Methodology
    Brief description of results
    Conclusions
    Implications
	8

Individual evidence table
    Evidence is categorized correctly
    Results displayed are accurate
    Limitations are listed
    Degree of support for the decision-making of evidence is accurate
	8

Evidence summary table
    Evidence is accurately summarized
    Practice recommendations are thorough
    Conclusions are based on the evidence presented
	9

Oral presentation	3
APA format is accurately used, and appendices are complete	2
(points could be deducted)	
TOTAL POINTS	**30**

FIGURE 1.4 Grading rubric for baccalaureate-level EBP project.

DISCUSSION BOARD QUESTIONS

Discussion board questions are a great way to engage students in EBP. Some discussion board questions appropriate to a baccalaureate-level course may include:

1. What do you think is the most important aspect of EBP in healthcare? Why is it critical for healthcare professionals to integrate research findings into their practice?

2. How do different types of research (qualitative vs. quantitative, systematic reviews vs. randomized controlled trials) contribute to EBP? Which do you think is most valuable in informing clinical decisions, and why?

3. How can healthcare leaders and organizations foster an environment that encourages EBP?

4. How does EBP support patient-centered care? Can you provide an example where a treatment or intervention might be based on evidence but might not align with a patient's values or preferences? How should healthcare professionals address such situations?

5. When reviewing research for EBP, what factors do you think are most important in determining the quality of the evidence?

6. Can you think of a specific instance where interdisciplinary collaboration might enhance the use of evidence-based practices? How would you encourage collaboration in a clinical setting?

PART 2
GRADUATE EDUCATION

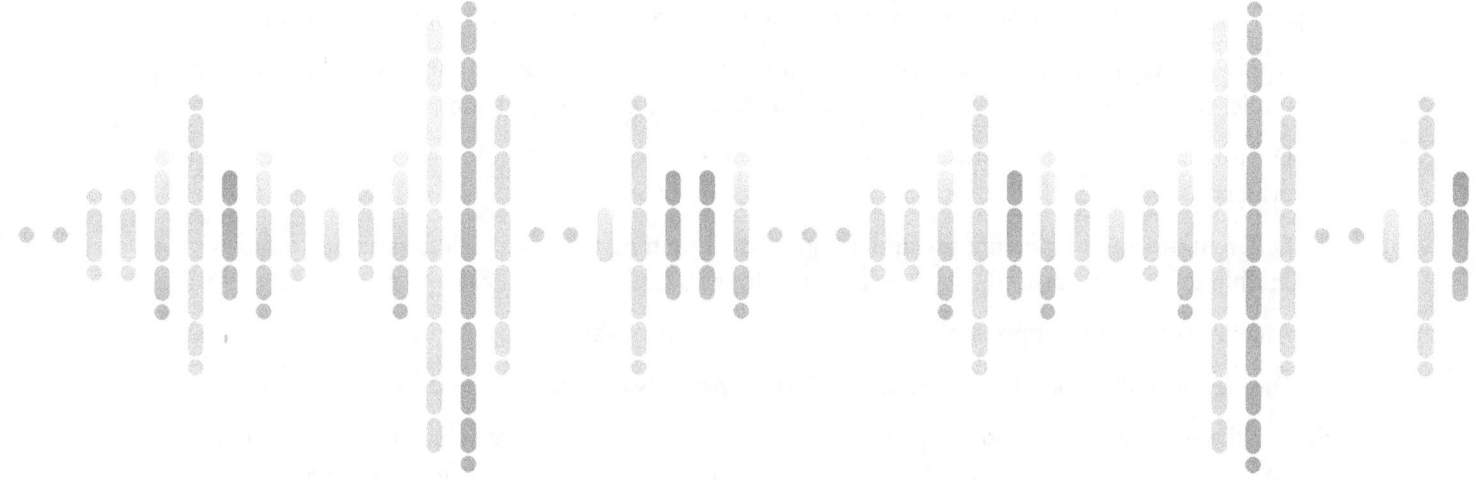

MASTER'S EDUCATION TEACHING GUIDE

The American Association of Colleges of Nursing's (AACN) *Essentials of Master's Education in Nursing* states that master's education must prepare the graduate to translate evidence into practice (AACN, 2011). In addition, accrediting agencies such as the Joint Commission and Magnet Recognition Program® have incorporated research and evidence-based practice (EBP) as necessary components of nursing practice for organizations to ensure healthcare excellence.

Similar to undergraduate programs in nursing, the master's program should integrate the EBP paradigm throughout the entire curriculum rather than limiting it to one or two courses. While undergraduates focus on foundational scholarship for practice, master's students are trained to apply new knowledge and translate it into practice. They use the same process as undergraduate students, but the expected outcomes of the course requirements are at a higher level. Additionally, while undergraduates are expected to develop an EBP question and critique an individual article related to that topic, master's students are required to assess the state of the science on a topic related to their practice specialty or an area of interest. The diverse backgrounds and abilities of incoming students present a challenge in graduate education. Some students matriculate with a recent research course and a thorough understanding of EBP basics, while others may need a refresher or an introduction to the basic content of EBP. All graduate research courses should emphasize translating research into practice settings.

Application of Research to Practice Course

One example of a master's level course is Application of Research to Practice. This essential core research course prepares students to apply the best available evidence into practice as they serve in advanced-level roles in healthcare organizations. The course includes a review of the research process (including theoretical framework, research design, and analysis); research critique; rating and synthesizing the strength of evidence; decision-making for practice; and research translation opportunities (outcomes, research evaluation, quality improvement, cost-effectiveness analysis), measurement, ethics, and types of organizational change. Although some of this material would have been covered at the undergraduate level, the emphasis in the master's course is on applying the concepts to evaluating and translating evidence related to practice.

Course Objectives

The objectives for the Application of Research to Practice course for the master's nursing student are:

1. Apply knowledge from the sciences to the advanced practice of nursing through utilization of an EBP model to answer a clinical, administrative, or education nursing question.
2. Demonstrate advanced knowledge of the research process and research designs through critique of evidence.
3. Differentiate among nursing research designs by examining their principles, variables, validity, sampling methods, procedures, strengths and limitations, and identification of knowledge gaps.
4. Analyze the various approaches to the measurement of variables.
5. Discuss the collection of data and the statistical methods used to analyze data.
6. Use the research process to address problems within areas of advanced clinical nursing practice and nursing systems by synthesizing the state of knowledge on a specific topic and recommending strategies to test interventions for improvement.

Learning Activities

Among many course requirements, two learning activities focus specifically on EBP skills and knowledge: a group research critique and an integrative review.

Group Research Critique

The group research critique requires students to demonstrate the ability to critically evaluate a research paper based on their knowledge of the research process and information on elements of a critique that they learned in class. For this assignment, students are divided into groups. Each group reads the assigned article(s) before the class session, with one of the articles designated for each group to present. The students use the appropriate Johns Hopkins Evidence-Based Practice (JHEBP) appraisal tools to analyze each article. Each group will present the article they read and provide a critique based on the appraisal checklist. The other groups, having also read that article, are allowed time to ask questions or provide comments.

Questions to consider may include (many may come from the appraisal tools):

1. What is the study's purpose?
2. For this study, define "cases" and "controls."
3. Is the study prospective or retrospective?
4. What statistical analyses were applied to the study data?
5. What are the clinical implications of the study findings?
6. Was the literature review comprehensive?

7. What were the study variables? Were they clearly defined?
8. How were the independent and dependent variables measured?
9. Were the measurement instruments reliable and valid?
10. Can the results be generalized?

Integrative Review

The second key assignment for the course is the integrative review. This paper is designed to reflect the student's ability to evaluate and synthesize current and relevant knowledge providing the state of evidence on a specific nursing issue. The assignment requires the student to conduct an exhaustive literature search, critically appraise the current evidence on the identified nursing issue, synthesize that evidence, and develop a plan to implement evidence-based recommendations from the evidence review (see Figure 2.1). In addition to the paper, students are required to fill out and submit the Individual Evidence Summary Tool (Appendix G2 in *Johns Hopkins Evidence-Based Practice for Nurses and Healthcare Professionals: Model & Guidelines*, 5th Edition) and the Summary, Synthesis, & Best-Evidence Recommendations Tool (Appendix H in the textbook). Students submit the paper in two parts so that they can receive feedback on their definition of the clinical problem and their search strategy. They review the literature and make recommendations in the second part of the paper.

Students are encouraged to choose topics for the integrative review that are in their specialty area or of clinical interest.

Integration of EBP Into Master's Clinical Courses

Identifying, using, and evaluating evidence related to practice, including standards of care (guidelines and protocols), is a focus of master's degree clinical courses. Students search various sources of evidence for current practice guidelines and are encouraged to download them to their electronic devices. During the weekly clinical conferences, students present and discuss relevant findings, including evaluation of use in their practice environments.

The use and evaluation of evidence in the clinical courses are not confined to the direct-care clinical courses. For example, health systems management students may review and evaluate the evidence used in the recommendations from the Institute of Medicine reports or position statements written by professional organizations, such as the American Nurses Association or the American Organization of Nurse Executives.

Master's Level Scholarly Project

In addition to the core research course, graduate students may be required to write an article to submit for publication or develop a poster for display. The purpose of the assignment is to investigate a complex clinical problem. Students are expected to synthesize and integrate knowledge gained from current and previous master's level coursework and apply that knowledge to a clinical problem by utilizing the best available scientific evidence. Projects may be developed over three academic semesters. In the first semester, the students may develop a problem statement on a topic of interest. In the second semester, the students may review the literature on this topic. In the final semester, the students may develop and present a poster on their project. The poster reflects and builds upon the students' clinical questions and problem statements developed in the first semester. It also builds upon the evidence-based review of the second semester's literature, evaluating the literature's strengths and implications.

PART I (FIVE-PAGE LIMIT, INCLUDING ABSTRACT, EXCLUDING REFERENCES): 10 POINTS TOTAL

Title (one page) and abstract (one page, double-spaced) **(1 pt)**

- Title: The title reflects the variables and population.
- Abstract: The abstract includes information about the problem, background, and purpose of the paper.

Introduction **(8 pts)**

- The problem and rationale are clear.
- The purpose of the paper is explicitly stated.
- The introduction presents a case for the need to study the topic and its relationship to nursing.
- All major concepts are introduced and defined.
- The search strategy, keywords, inclusion criteria, and number and types of evidence reviewed are included and adequately described.

Organization/Formatting **(1 pt)**

- There is a logical flow of ideas and proper grammar and spelling.
- The paper, including citations and references, uses APA format correctly throughout.

PART II (10-PAGE LIMIT, EXCLUDING ABSTRACT, REFERENCES, AND APPENDICES)

1. An abstract—with a conclusion related to the state of the science—has been added.
2. The state of the science on the nursing issue is described with sources of evidence critically reviewed and synthesized. The evidence is summarized in the JHEBP Individual Evidence Summary Tool.
3. The strengths and limitations of the current evidence are described. The evidence base for practice change is clearly supported, or the identified gap in evidence is compelling and significant.
4. Implications for nursing research/practice/policy are identified and linked to the level of evidence from the preceding synthesis of literature.
5. Recommendations for translating evidence to practice or initiation of further research are identified and linked to the level of evidence from the preceding synthesis of literature. This should include a feasible plan for implementation of EBP, an identification of key impacted groups and an appropriate interdisciplinary team to assemble, and a brief plan for outcome analysis, including independent and dependent variables and a method of statistical analysis.

FIGURE 2.1 Integrative review paper guidelines and grading rubric.

DISCUSSION BOARD QUESTIONS

Discussion board questions are a great way to engage students in EBP. Some questions appropriate for a master's level course may include:

1. How would you address potential conflicts between evidence-based recommendations and institutional practices or policies that may not align with the latest evidence?

2. Systematic reviews and meta-analyses are often considered the gold standard in EBP. What are the key strengths and limitations of relying on these types of studies when making clinical decisions?

3. EBP emphasizes the integration of the best available research with clinical expertise. How do you balance the use of research evidence with clinical judgment, particularly in complex or novel patient cases where evidence may be limited or inconclusive?

4. How do you navigate situations where research evidence may conflict with clinical experience or a patient's preferences, and how can this be addressed in an ethical and patient-centered way?

5. Large healthcare organizations often encounter systemic barriers to implementing EBP (e.g., resource constraints, staff resistance, or organizational culture). What strategies can leaders adopt to overcome these barriers and promote the uptake of EBP across multidisciplinary teams?

6. The ultimate goal of EBP is to improve patient outcomes. How do you measure and evaluate the impact of EBP interventions on patient outcomes in your clinical area, and what are some of the challenges in assessing these outcomes?

7. In your experience or observation, what are the barriers to successful interdisciplinary collaboration in EBP, and how can these be mitigated?

8. In EBP, it is crucial to consider the cultural context of the patient population. How do you ensure that evidence-based interventions are culturally appropriate and effective for diverse patient populations, and what challenges might arise when research findings do not adequately address cultural factors?

DOCTORAL EDUCATION TEACHING GUIDE

Doctoral education in nursing today follows two distinct degree paths: Doctor of Philosophy (PhD) and Doctor of Nursing Practice (DNP). Both programs contribute to the expansion of nursing knowledge and the development of specialized skills, each with a distinct focus. PhD programs emphasize the generation of new knowledge through rigorous research, while DNP programs concentrate on translating this knowledge into practice to solve real-world healthcare challenges. Importantly, both degree paths focus specifically on advancing the discipline of nursing and require students to engage in critical evaluation of the existing body of evidence.

At the doctoral level, students are challenged to critically evaluate and synthesize evidence not only from nursing but also from a wide range of sciences and other disciplines. This broad scope of evidence is essential for answering key nursing-related questions and solving complex practice problems. Given the expansive and diverse nature of this evidence, doctoral students can greatly benefit from structured frameworks like the one offered in *Johns Hopkins Evidence-Based Practice for Nurses and Healthcare Professionals: Model & Guidelines,* 5th Edition. This model supports students in organizing, appraising, and synthesizing evidence systematically, ensuring a logical, integrative approach to developing solutions.

PhD education focuses primarily on research, which is the discovery of new knowledge. Students are prepared to ask critical questions about nursing and healthcare issues where current evidence is insufficient or lacking. Throughout PhD education, students acquire an expert understanding of the theories, methods, and analytical approaches relevant to the field of nursing. The research is characterized by methodological rigor, including precise design, control of extraneous variables, reliable and valid measurement tools, and thorough evaluation of the evidence. PhD students engage in the creation of foundational knowledge that serves as a basis for future inquiry and application. The AACN Position Statement on Nursing Research can be found at https://www.aacnnursing.org/Portals/0/PDFs/Position-Statements/Nursing-Research.pdf.

DNP education emphasizes the application of knowledge to improve practice outcomes and prepares nurse leaders at the highest level of nursing practice. Driven by a spirit of inquiry, DNP students focus on solving existing practice problems by implementing evidence-based interventions, with a primary goal of improving patient outcomes. DNP-prepared nurses are uniquely equipped to translate research into practice, ensuring that the cutting-edge discoveries are effectively applied in real-world clinical settings. DNP students actively engage in addressing practice problems by applying or translating the latest research discoveries into clinical practice. DNP students ensure the fidelity of evidence translation, meticulously monitor outcomes, and assess the sustainability of the interventions they implement. This hands-on approach, while carefully structured, stands apart from the work of PhD students by focusing directly on real-world application and the improvement of healthcare delivery systems. DNP students navigate the complexities of healthcare practice environments, where confounding variables are prevalent, and commonly rely on data collected for other purposes to evaluate the success of their interventions. By focusing on the translation of evidence into practice, DNP students play a crucial role in advancing the quality of healthcare, ensuring that patient care is grounded in the best available evidence. DNP students are instrumental in translating evidence into practice while navigating a complex real-world environment that is grounded in clinical operations, clinical expertise, and EBP. The AACN Position Statement on the Practice Doctorate in Nursing can be found at https://www.aacnnursing.org/our-initiatives/education-practice/doctor-of-nursing-practice/position-statement.

A PRIMER ON EVIDENCE-BASED PRACTICE

According to Bissett et al. (2025), EBP is a critical competency for all healthcare professionals across the care continuum. EBP is mandated by professional standards, regulatory bodies, and healthcare insurers and is a cornerstone of high-reliability organizations, fostering a culture of safety and excellence.

By integrating research into practice, EBP enables healthcare organizations to meet the quadruple aim: improving patient care, improving population health, reducing costs, and enhancing the well-being of healthcare providers (Migliore et al., 2020). EBP ensures that care decisions are based on the best available evidence, promoting quality, consistency, and patient-centered outcomes.

For doctoral nursing students, particularly those with limited exposure to EBP, the JHEBP Model for Nurses and Healthcare Professionals serves as an invaluable resource. This model offers a structured and comprehensive framework to guide the integration of research evidence into clinical and organizational decision-making. As stated in the 5th edition of *Johns Hopkins Evidence-Based Practice for Nurses and Healthcare Professionals: Model & Guidelines*, "The PET (Practice Question, Evidence, and Translation) process shown in the EBP model provides a systematic approach for developing a practice question, finding the best evidence, and translating the best evidence into practice" (Bissett et al., 2025, pp. 24–25). By utilizing this model, students are empowered to critically appraise and apply evidence systematically, enhancing their ability to lead evidence-based initiatives and improve care outcomes within their respective healthcare environments.

The domains, competencies, and concepts presented in *Essentials: Core Competencies for Professional Nursing Education* (AACN, 2021) provide a solid foundation for curriculum design and program evaluation, ensuring consistent outcomes for graduates. Part 5 of this guide features a sample DNP scholarly project curriculum outline aligned with the AACN *Essentials* (AACN, 2021). The framework utilized to inform the curriculum outline included the JHEBP model PET Pathway (Bissett et al., 2025) and the framework from Implementing the EBP Competencies in Academic Settings: EBP Integration in Graduate Programs, by Melnyk and Fineout-Overholt (2019).

The curriculum outline fully integrates the tools provided by the JHEBP model to guide doctoral students through the EBP process in a systematic and structured way. These tools are specifically designed to help students critically appraise and apply research evidence, ensuring they move through each phase of their scholarly projects with clarity and purpose. By utilizing the JHEBP model's comprehensive framework, the curriculum not only aligns with the core competencies outlined in the AACN *Essentials* but also empowers students to develop the skills needed to lead evidence-based initiatives effectively. This structured approach ensures that students are well-prepared to translate research into practice, improve patient outcomes, and contribute meaningfully to healthcare systems.

In the next sections, which refer to specific chapters in the textbook, faculty will guide doctoral students through the essential steps of gathering, appraising, and synthesizing evidence to ensure their EBP projects are built on a solid foundation of best practices and reliable data.

FACULTY GUIDANCE IN DEVELOPING EFFECTIVE EBP QUESTIONS FOR DOCTORAL PROJECTS

In the JHEBP model, faculty play a critical role in guiding students through the practice question phase. This phase lays the foundation for impactful EBP projects by ensuring that students thoroughly explore the problem, develop well-defined problem statements, and craft answerable questions that align with clinical needs and organizational priorities. These efforts reflect the AACN *Essentials* (2021) focus on inquiry, leadership, and EBP.

EBP: Past, Present, and Future (Chapter 1)

EBP fosters critical thinking and continuous learning, enabling effective, efficient, and equitable patient care. The faculty must highlight how recent challenges, like the COVID-19 pandemic, demonstrate the need for rapid evidence appraisal. Additionally, faculty should emphasize that while technologies like artificial intelligence can enhance EBP, skilled clinicians are essential for interpreting and validating evidence, ensuring sound decision-making and ethical practice.

The Johns Hopkins Evidence-Based Practice (JHEBP) Model for Nurses and Healthcare Professionals (HCPs) Process Overview (Chapter 2)

The JHEBP model's 16-step PET process ensures rigorous, systematic EBP. Faculty guide students through each phase, promoting interprofessional collaboration, mentorship, and alignment with organizational priorities for sustainable project outcomes. This structured guidance ensures sustainable project outcomes and fosters the professional competencies required by the AACN *Essentials*.

Practice Question Phase: The Problem (Chapter 3)

The AACN *Essentials* (2021) emphasize problem-solving and inquiry, which align closely with the practice question phase. Faculty should encourage students to thoroughly explore the problem using tools like root cause analyses, data gathering, and interprofessional collaboration to refine the problem statement. A clear, well-defined statement motivates action and sets the stage for an effective EBP question.

Crafting Effective Problem Statements

Faculty guide students to fully explore and describe the problem. This may include conducting a root cause analysis, using the 5-Whys technique, fishbone diagramming, or concept mapping. This approach ensures students identify the actual problem and, thus, discover optimal solutions. Key guiding questions include:

- What is the local problem?
- Why is it important, and what are the consequences if unresolved?
- What is the current practice?
- What data supports the problem's existence?

By aligning their guidance with the AACN *Essentials* (2021), faculty help students develop the critical competencies needed for evidence-based inquiry and leadership. Through structured mentorship, faculty ensure students master the skills to develop high-quality EBP questions, positioning them to address complex healthcare challenges and drive meaningful, sustainable improvements in patient care.

Practice Question Phase: The EBP Question (Chapter 4)

The practice question phase is the initial step of the PET process, where EBP projects emerge from questions or problems needing further exploration. The practice phase, the "P" in the PET process, includes three critical steps:

- Explore and describe the problem

- Develop the problem statement
- Write the EBP question

These steps form the foundation of a well-defined practice question that lays the groundwork for efficient evidence-based inquiry and guides the next phase of the process, the evidence phase (the "E" in the PET process), toward solution development. The translation phase, the "T" in the PET process, is the final step. This component ensures that evidence-based recommendations are evaluated for fit, feasibility, and readiness, driving meaningful improvements in outcomes, safety, and healthcare policy. Faculty play an essential role in mentoring students through these steps, ensuring alignment with the competencies outlined in the AACN *Essentials* (2021), which emphasize inquiry, leadership, and evidence-based decision-making.

Evolving the EBP Question Framework: Aligning With the AACN *Essentials* (2021)

As the JHEBP model has evolved, the traditional terms "background" and "foreground" have been reconsidered, leading to a new approach that better aligns with the needs of its users. The updated JHEBP model (Bissett et al., 2025) introduces fill-in-the-blank structures and suggested terms for constructing EBP questions, moving away from the constraints of the PICO format. While the PICO tool remains valuable for some in focusing their efforts, it has been found to hinder the inquiry process for doctoral students by encouraging premature focus on a specific solution. This often skews the search for evidence, prioritizing validation of the chosen intervention rather than facilitating an objective discovery of the most effective solution through rigorous evaluation. Faculty play a key role in mentoring students to explore local problems thoroughly, fostering critical thinking, leadership, and alignment with the AACN *Essentials* (2021).

Informing the AACN *Essentials* (2021)

This revised questioning framework aligns with the AACN *Essentials* (2021) by fostering inquiry, critical thinking, and data-driven decision-making. The *Essentials* emphasize developing advanced problem-solving skills and leadership competencies—attributes cultivated through this updated EBP approach. Faculty play a key role in helping students engage in open inquiry, enabling them to objectively assess evidence and align their projects with clinical and organizational priorities.

New Questioning Framework

To overcome the limitations of the traditional PICO format, the JHEBP model (Dang et al., 2021) adopted a revised EBP framework designed to encourage a more thorough and open-ended inquiry. This updated format prompts students to identify key concepts important to the problem without spending unnecessary time trying to fit concepts into a question structure. For example, students just starting work on a problem will often not have an intervention or an outcome identified to complete the I and O of the PICO.

A well-defined problem statement is essential to guide the next steps in the EBP process. Faculty ensure that students develop meaningful, answerable questions that align with clinical priorities and institutional goals, preparing them to implement sustainable, evidence-based solutions.

Broad vs. Intervention Questions

Faculty should guide students to begin with a broad best-practice question, especially when unfamiliar with the topic or potential interventions. Although not always required, this approach ensures that intervention questions are informed by current evidence, aligning with best practices and meeting the AACN *Essentials* (2021) competencies for inquiry and advanced practice.

A broad DNP question typically explores a general concept, issue, or phenomenon related to nursing practice, while a DNP intervention question focuses on a specific action or strategy intended to bring about change or improvement in patient care or healthcare systems.

Broad question example: "What are the best strategies for nurse-led quality improvement initiatives in acute care settings?"

This question is exploratory and examines a general relationship rather than testing a specific intervention.

Intervention question example: "According to the evidence, in hospitalized inpatient adults (65 and older), what is the impact of the implementation of an EBP structured fall prevention protocol, compared to standard care, on the incidence of falls over six months?"

Evaluating Project Relevance

Faculty support is essential in helping students assess whether their project aligns with organizational strategic goals, as projects that address institutional priorities are more likely to receive time, resources, and engagement from impacted groups. This aligns with the AACN *Essentials* (2021) by fostering leadership and collaboration.

Crafting High-Quality Questions

Faculty should emphasize the importance of spending time on question development, as well-constructed questions streamline the EBP process and reduce the risk of setbacks. Spending time on question refinement ensures a smooth EBP process, reduces obstacles, and promotes outcomes that align with both the JHEBP framework and the AACN *Essentials* (2021) competencies for effective, evidence-based healthcare leadership.

FACULTY MENTORING FOR LEADERSHIP AND COLLABORATION

The Interprofessional Team (Chapter 5)

In the JHEBP model, interprofessional collaboration is essential for the successful implementation of EBP projects. Faculty play a key role in mentoring students to build, lead, and manage diverse teams, ensuring that the project benefits from the varied knowledge and expertise of healthcare professionals. This collaborative approach strengthens evidence-based interventions and drives sustainable improvements in healthcare outcomes.

Faculty guide students in selecting core team members, appointing effective leaders, and identifying partners essential to the project's success. Encouraging students to engage team members early ensures that multiple perspectives shape the project from the start.

Facilitating Collaboration and Problem-Solving

Faculty help students foster strong teamwork by promoting open communication and shared goals, while also developing strategies to address challenges such as miscommunication, role ambiguity, or competing priorities.

Maintaining Engagement and Accountability

To keep projects on track, faculty assist students in using tools such as a Gantt chart and a Work Breakdown Structure. These tools support consistent engagement, ensuring that the team remains aligned and accountable throughout the project (Verzuh, 2021).

Through the recommendations provided in Chapter 5, faculty can help students develop essential leadership skills to form and manage effective interprofessional teams. This guidance equips students to navigate challenges, maintain accountability, and foster collaboration, thus ensuring that EBP projects lead to improved patient care and health outcomes.

FACULTY GUIDANCE FOR THE EVIDENCE PHASE FOR DOCTORAL STUDENTS

As faculty guide students through the JHEBP model, it is essential to emphasize that searching, reviewing, and appraising the literature are foundational steps in developing informed, evidence-based solutions. As facilitators, faculty play a critical role in guiding students through this phase to ensure they develop precise, well-framed questions that guide the evidence phase effectively. This phase ensures that students understand what constitutes credible evidence, how to gather it effectively, and how to critically assess its relevance and quality to support their EBP projects.

Key Steps in the Evidence Phase

1. **Introduction to Evidence (Chapter 6):** Faculty should introduce students to the concept of evidence and the various types they will encounter, such as primary research, systematic reviews, and expert opinions. It is also important to highlight recent updates to the JHEBP model to ensure that students align their projects with current evidence-based healthcare practices.

2. **Evidence Search and Screening (Chapter 7):** Guide students on when, where, and how to conduct literature searches. Encourage the use of pre-appraised evidence when possible but prepare them to perform comprehensive searches for more complex inquiries. Remind students to be mindful of biases during their search, which could skew results toward a specific intervention. Figure 2.2 highlights a sample course assignment around searching and corresponding rubric.

3. **Appraising the Evidence (Chapter 8):** Support students as they learn to evaluate the quality and applicability of evidence. Teach them how to tailor appraisal techniques to different study types, ensuring that they select the most reliable evidence to guide their practice decisions. This phase prepares them to summarize and synthesize their findings into actionable recommendations.

By fostering a methodical and unbiased approach to literature work, faculty play a vital role in preparing students to navigate the evidence phase effectively. Through this guidance, students become proficient in the critical steps of gathering, screening, and appraising literature, equipping them to generate meaningful, evidence-based solutions that improve healthcare outcomes.

GRADING RUBRIC: SEARCH STRATEGY ASSIGNMENT

CRITERIA	EXEMPLARY (4 POINTS)	PROFICIENT (3 POINTS)	BASIC (2 POINTS)	NEEDS IMPROVEMENT (1 POINT)
Search Strategy	Clearly articulated search strategy that is logical, thorough, and well-structured. The strategy includes specific details about the process and rationale.	Adequately defined search strategy that is logical and mostly clear but may lack some detail or thoroughness.	Basic search strategy is presented but lacks logical flow or detail and may be vague in parts.	Poorly defined or unclear search strategy with little to no logical structure.
Database and Source Selection	Uses a variety of appropriate databases and resources that are highly relevant to the topic. Rationale for database selection is clearly explained.	Selects appropriate databases with some variety. Rationale for selection is adequate but lacks full detail.	Uses limited or somewhat inappropriate sources and lacks clear rationale for selection.	Uses few or inappropriate databases/sources without any rationale or relevance to the topic.
Keyword Selection and Boolean Logic	Comprehensive and relevant keywords are chosen, with effective use of Boolean operators, truncation, and filters.	Keywords are mostly relevant, and Boolean logic is used adequately but may lack variety or precision.	Uses limited or partially relevant keywords and minimal use of Boolean operators or filters.	Inadequate keyword selection with ineffective or no use of Boolean logic and filters.
Evaluation of Sources	Critically evaluates sources for credibility, relevance, and quality. Includes detailed criteria for selection and rejection.	Evaluates sources based on credibility and relevance, but criteria are not fully detailed.	Source evaluation is minimal, with limited criteria for credibility and relevance assessment.	Little to no evaluation of source quality, credibility, or relevance.

| Documentation and Organization | The assignment is well-organized, with clear headings, a logical flow, and accurate APA (or other specified style) citations. | Generally organized and follows a logical structure. Minor citation or formatting errors. | Some organizational issues and frequent citation errors. | Disorganized with poor structure and many citation errors. |

FIGURE 2.2 Evaluation of search strategy rubric.

Summary, Synthesis, and Best-Evidence Recommendations (Chapter 9)

The Individual Evidence Summary Tool—Appendix G2 in the textbook—can be helpful as a template to organize the large and complex body of information relevant to the research question or practice problem. Because of the tremendous variability in the nature and the quality of evidence available to drive practice improvement (opinion statements, institutional guidelines, case studies, and research), the model is particularly useful for DNP students. The Summary, Synthesis, & Best-Evidence Recommendations Tool, Appendix H in the textbook, can aid doctoral students in managing the rating of individual studies and items of evidence. This tool allows students to combine all pieces of applicable evidence and synthesize that material.

Doctoral students, like practicing nurses, need to be able to discriminate levels of quality and rigor across disparate documents and to present the findings reported in this context. The students need to create a logical argument for the strategy proposed to address the clinical problem. Synthesis of evidence based on an assessment of quantity, consistency, and applicability is key for the students to make an overall recommendation and the critical decision about which evidence should be translated to solve the practice problem in a particular setting. The Individual Evidence Summary Tool helps manage this complex assignment.

Chapter 9 of the textbook emphasizes the critical steps in the evidence phase focused on appraising, organizing, and synthesizing evidence to develop best-evidence recommendations. Faculty guide students in using methods like the "rule of rows and columns" (Garrard, 2014, in Bissett et al., 2025) to systematically compile and analyze evidence for clear interpretation.

This phase covers Steps 7–10 of the EBP process (refer to Chapter 9, Box 9.1 in the textbook), including summarizing, organizing, and synthesizing findings to form actionable recommendations. Key tools such as the JHEBP Pre-Appraised Evidence Summary Tool (Appendix G1), Individual Evidence Summary Tool (Appendix G2), and Summary, Synthesis, & Best-Evidence Recommendations Tool (Appendix H) help facilitate this process.

Key Areas of Focus for Faculty:

1. Evidence summary: Encourage students to collate information objectively without personal interpretation
2. Organization: Assist students in sorting data into meaningful categories for easier analysis
3. Synthesis: Guide students in synthesizing evidence to identify patterns and generate new insights

Key Steps for Faculty (Box 9.1):

4. Conduct best-evidence search and appraisal
5. Conduct targeted evidence search or conduct exhaustive search and screening
6. Appraise the evidence
7. Summarize the evidence
8. Organize the data
9. Synthesize the findings
10. Record best-practice recommendations

By following these steps, faculty ensure that students develop objective, well-organized, and synthesized evidence summaries that lead to strong, evidence-based recommendations. These recommendations not only lay the foundation for successful practice changes but also align with the AACN *Essentials* (2021), helping students meet key competencies in EBP, critical thinking, and leadership.

FACULTY GUIDANCE FOR THE TRANSLATION, IMPLEMENTATION, AND DISSEMINATION PHASES FOR DOCTORAL STUDENTS

In the JHEBP model, the final stages of the PET process—translation, implementation, and dissemination—are essential for translating evidence into practice and driving lasting change. Faculty play a key role in mentoring students through these phases to ensure successful execution and impactful outcomes.

Translation Phase: Translation (Chapter 10)

The translation phase focuses on applying evidence-based recommendations using frameworks like the TRIP model. Faculty guide students in setting goals, timelines, and success measures, while helping them identify and overcome barriers. Sustainability planning is emphasized to ensure that practice changes persist beyond project closure. Effective communication and collaboration across teams further support smooth implementation.

Effective translation of evidence into practice requires the assessment of several key metrics and organizational considerations to ensure successful implementation. Translating evidence is not merely about determining whether there is a need for change but involves an in-depth analysis of various criteria that influence the recommendation for a practice change. Chapter 10 of *Johns Hopkins Evidence-Based Practice for Nurses and Healthcare Professionals: Model & Guidelines*, 5th Edition, outlines this process, emphasizing the importance of evaluating organizational readiness to avoid potential failures that can waste time and resources.

The process of translation must account for factors such as safety risk, fit, feasibility, and acceptability within the specific organizational context. These metrics enable facilitators to assess the feasibility and timing of an evidence-based intervention, ensuring it is both suitable and optimally timed for successful implementation. This evaluation process is essential for determining the intervention's potential impact and aligning it with the specific needs and readiness of the target setting. Faculty will guide teams in leveraging these metrics to make informed decisions regarding which practices to implement and when to achieve the most sustainable change.

The final step is the translation of the evidence into practice. Chapter 11 in the textbook provides a framework for guiding this implementation process into practice. The translation process is outlined detailing practical steps to help navigate from evidence appraisal to actual practice change.

Translation Phase: Implementation (Chapter 11)

Chapter 11 outlines the critical role of structured approaches in translating EBP into actionable, sustainable changes within healthcare organizations. Chapter 11 highlights the TRIP (Translating Research Into Practice) model as a foundational framework that guides the EBP team through the process of implementing evidence-based recommendations. The knowledge of various frameworks is important for faculty to include when educating on the JHEBP model. Translation frameworks may be introduced early within a DNP program, potentially as part of an initial project course—toward the end of the first course, at the beginning of the second, or as a stand-alone one-credit course. This approach ensures that students gain foundational knowledge in applying translation science, equipping them to integrate evidence into practice effectively as they progress through the program.

Ongoing Considerations: Communication and Dissemination (Chapter 12)

Dissemination is critical for advancing healthcare and aligns with professional ethics, such as those outlined by the American Nurses Association and American Medical Association. Faculty mentor students in selecting appropriate channels—such as publications or presentations—to share findings, enhancing knowledge and catalyzing change. Students bring valuable clinical insight to their projects, combining practical experience with evidence-based recommendations to advocate for patients, staff, and populations. Figure 2.3 provides a basic outline for an EBP project dissemination paper.

RUBRIC FOR EBP PAPER

CRITERIA	EXEMPLARY (90–100 POINTS)	PROFICIENT (80–89 POINTS)	SATISFACTORY (70–79 POINTS)	NEEDS IMPROVEMENT (60–69 POINTS)	UNSATISFACTORY (0–59 POINTS)
Introduction & Problem Identification (20 points)	Clearly defines the clinical problem and its significance to practice; includes a compelling introduction that engages the reader. Demonstrates an in-depth understanding of the problem's impact on healthcare.	Adequately defines the clinical problem with relevant details on significance to practice. Introduction is clear, though may lack some depth.	Defines the problem, though lacks depth or clarity in connecting it to practice. Introduction is basic.	Minimally defines the problem; lacks detail and context in connection to practice. Introduction is unclear.	Fails to define the problem effectively; no connection to clinical practice is established.

continues

RUBRIC FOR EBP PAPER (CONT.)

CRITERIA	EXEMPLARY (90–100 POINTS)	PROFICIENT (80–89 POINTS)	SATISFACTORY (70–79 POINTS)	NEEDS IMPROVEMENT (60–69 POINTS)	UNSATISFACTORY (0–59 POINTS)
Literature Review & Evidence Synthesis (25 points)	Thoroughly reviews and synthesizes high-quality, relevant evidence. Demonstrates a clear, critical understanding of literature with synthesis that supports the problem and initiatives chosen.	Reviews relevant literature, though synthesis may lack depth. Evidence generally supports the problem and initiatives.	Basic review of literature with limited synthesis. Evidence lacks clear alignment with the problem and initiatives.	Minimal review of literature, with unclear synthesis and limited relevance to the problem.	Lacks a literature review or fails to provide relevant or credible evidence.
Practice Initiative(s) Selection & Rationale (20 points)	Provides a thorough description and rationale for selected practice initiative(s). Clearly aligns initiatives with EBP to address the clinical problem effectively.	Adequately describes the selected initiative(s) with some rationale; aligns with EBP and addresses the clinical problem.	Describes initiative(s), though rationale and alignment with EBP are unclear or insufficiently detailed.	Minimally describes initiative(s); lacks clear rationale or EBP alignment with the clinical problem.	Fails to describe initiative(s) effectively or lacks rationale and alignment with EBP.
Implementation Plan & Methods (15 points)	Clearly articulates a well-organized, feasible implementation plan with detailed methods. Methods are aligned with EBP and clearly support the objectives.	Provides an organized implementation plan with relevant methods; some alignment with EBP is evident.	Implementation plan and methods are basic and lack some alignment with EBP.	Minimally developed implementation plan and methods, with limited alignment with EBP.	Fails to provide a coherent implementation plan or methods aligned with EBP.
Implications for Practice (10 points)	Thoroughly discusses the implications of the practice initiative on clinical practice, including potential impacts on patient care and outcomes.	Discusses implications for practice, though may lack some depth in exploring impacts on care and outcomes.	Briefly mentions implications for practice but lacks depth and clear connection to outcomes.	Minimally addresses implications for practice, with limited connection to patient care or outcomes.	Fails to address implications for practice.

Conclusion & Synthesis (5 points)	Provides a concise, insightful conclusion that synthesizes key points from the paper, reinforcing the importance of EBP in addressing the clinical problem.	Summarizes key points with adequate synthesis, though lacks some insight. Conclusion reinforces the importance of EBP.	Conclusion is basic, with limited synthesis of key points.	Conclusion minimally summarizes key points; lacks synthesis and connection to EBP.	Fails to provide a meaningful conclusion.
Writing Quality & APA Formatting (5 points)	Writing is clear, professional, and engaging with no grammatical errors. Consistently adheres to APA formatting guidelines.	Writing is clear and professional with minimal errors. Generally follows APA guidelines with minor issues.	Writing is understandable but lacks professionalism or contains multiple errors. APA formatting inconsistently applied.	Writing is unclear and contains frequent errors; APA formatting is minimally followed.	Writing is unclear with numerous errors; APA formatting is not followed.

Score Ranges

- **Exemplary** (90–100 points): Outstanding work, with thorough understanding and application of EBP principles. Exceeds expectations in organization, depth, and professional quality.
- **Proficient** (80–89 points): Competent work, showing adequate understanding and alignment with EBP. Meets course expectations.
- **Satisfactory** (70–79 points): Basic understanding demonstrated. Meets some criteria but lacks depth in analysis or synthesis.
- **Needs Improvement** (60–69 points): Limited understanding of EBP; multiple areas need improvement.
- **Unsatisfactory** (0–59 points): Does not meet the basic criteria for understanding or applying EBP.

FIGURE 2.3 Rubric for EBP paper.

Faculty support ensures students develop strong implementation strategies and sustainability plans. Encouraging dissemination helps students promote evidence-based care, inspire change, and contribute to professional growth. Faculty guidance through implementation and dissemination empowers students to translate evidence into practice, sustain improvements, and share their work to advance healthcare and patient outcomes.

PART 3
PROFESSIONAL DEVELOPMENT FOR HEALTHCARE ORGANIZATIONS

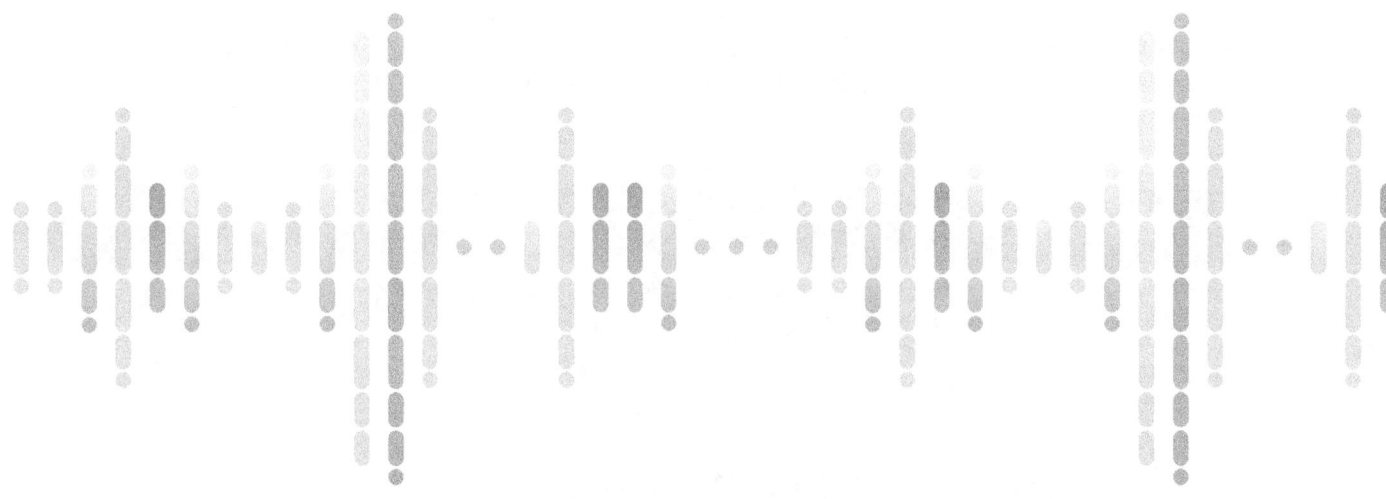

PROFESSIONAL DEVELOPMENT FACILITATOR GUIDE

Evidence-based practice (EBP) education within a healthcare organization aims to equip healthcare professionals with the knowledge and skills needed to translate best practice into the clinical setting. There is no "one size fits all" approach to developing an EBP education program, as each healthcare organization is unique, and a variety of strategies can be used to ensure EBP competency. This unit can be used as a step-by-step guide to help you develop a program that meets the needs of your specific healthcare organization.

BUILD AN EBP STEERING COMMITTEE

Developing an EBP education program across an organization is a major undertaking and requires proper planning, development, and commitment. It is highly recommended to develop the program with an EBP steering committee. As the name suggests, a steering committee will help "steer" or guide the program. This includes setting a strategic focus, making key decisions, communicating with relevant parties, and managing resources (Karlsen, 2020).

When building your steering committee, recruit people for the team that have system leadership and/or technical leadership (Institute for Healthcare Improvement, n.d.). People with system leadership have the authority to implement the program and obtain key resources. This includes senior management (e.g., chief nursing officers), middle management (e.g., directors of nursing), and first-line management (e.g., nurse managers). People with technical leadership have the knowledge and skills to build the program and make technical decisions. This includes inquiry and education experts, such as EBP, quality improvement, and research coordinators and nurse educators.

In addition to building a team with both system and technical leadership, you will also want your committee to be diverse. Healthcare is multifaceted, so your steering committee should be too! Including people with varied disciplines, experiences, and perspectives will help improve the problem-solving ability of the group, gain cross-discipline buy-in, ensure optimal use of resources, and, ultimately, lead to a more comprehensive and effective program (Newhouse & Spring, 2010).

Finally, you will want to consider the size of the committee. The size of a committee can significantly impact productivity. Committees that are too small may lack the necessary knowledge and expertise to ensure success of the program. On the other hand, committees that are too large may have difficulty communicating and collaborating. Ideally, steering committees are comprised of five to nine members; groups of this size tend to work more effectively and produce higher quality work (Lim & Klein, 2006; Mueller, 2012).

> **ADDITIONAL RESOURCES**
>
> Visit Hopkins.org/resources to download additional resources to support the development of an EBP steering committee at your organization, including a sample committee charter.

PERFORM LEARNING NEEDS ASSESSMENT

The next step in developing an EBP education program is to perform a learning needs assessment. A *learning needs assessment* is a structured process for identifying what knowledge, skills, and behaviors people need to learn (English & Kaufman, 1975). Taking the time to identify the learning needs of your staff upfront will help you design an EBP education program that is tailored to the needs of your organization. There are several ways to perform a learning needs assessment. Some of the more common methods are surveys, focus groups, and interviews.

Surveys

Staff surveys are one of the quickest and easiest ways to assess the learning needs of your staff. Staff surveys are a great option if you are limited on time and resources. To conduct a staff survey, it is essential that you use a survey tool that has been validated in your target population. For example, if you are aiming to understand the learning needs of your respiratory therapists (RTs), the survey questions should have been tested and proven to accurately reflect the learning needs of RTs.

You do not need to develop and validate a new survey tool. Several survey tools have been validated to assess EBP attitudes, behaviors, and skills, many of which have been validated in multiple healthcare disciplines (Landsverk et al., 2023). Some examples of validated survey tools include the EBP Inventory, Al Zoubi Questionnaire, EBP Process Assessment Scale (EBPPAS), Health Sciences EBP Questionnaire (HS-EBP), EBP Profile Questionnaire (EBP2), and the Instrument to Assess Evidence-Based Health (I-SABE; Al Zoubi et al., 2018; Fernandez-Dominguez et al., 2016; Kaper et al., 2015; McEvoy et al., 2010; Ruano et al., 2022; Rubin & Parrish, 2010).

Surveys can be administered either online or on paper. Online surveys are generally preferred because they are cheaper, quicker, easier, and more accurate. However, paper surveys may be preferred in rural and remote regions that may not have access to a reliable internet connection, or with staff that are not technology proficient.

If you choose to administer your survey online, several online survey platforms are available. Features vary by platform, including cost, design options, security, and ease of use. Some of the more popular platforms are Qualtrics, Microsoft Forms, Survey Monkey, and Alchemer.

Focus Groups

You can also use focus groups to assess the learning needs of your staff. Focus groups require more time and effort to implement than surveys but allow you to gain a more in-depth understanding of the learning needs of your staff.

To conduct a focus group, start by identifying someone to be the moderator or facilitator. This is typically someone from your EBP steering committee. The moderator is responsible for keeping the conversation on track and flowing organically, encouraging everyone to speak, and creating a comfortable environment (Onwuegbuzie et al., 2009).

Next, with the help of your EBP steering committee, develop a list of 8 to 10 questions or prompts for the moderator to use to guide the discussion (Centers for Disease Control and Prevention [CDC], 2018; Marczak & Sewell, n.d.). Avoid closed-ended questions that can be answered with "yes" or "no"; instead, use open-ended questions that encourage conversation. For example, instead of asking "Is EBP important to your practice?" ask "How does EBP influence your practice?"

Once you have your focus group planned, invite a small group of staff to participate. Each focus group should have between 6 and 12 participants, enough people to gather a variety of opinions, but not too many people that not everyone has a chance to talk (CDC, 2018; Onwuegbuzi et al., 2009). Each focus group should also be comprised of people with similar characteristics, such as occupation, education level, age, etc., so people feel comfortable sharing their honest opinions. For example, newer clinicians may not feel comfortable sharing their honest opinions and experiences if they are in the same group as their managers or supervisors.

Your focus group should last between one and two hours (CDC, 2018; Onwuegbuzi et al., 2009). Focus groups that last shorter than one hour typically do not have enough time to explore all questions in-depth, and focus groups that last longer than two hours tend to lose the interest of the group. Start by asking engagement or "ice breaker" questions that ease the group into discussion (University of Mississippi, 2005). For example, "What is EBP?" Once the group has warmed up to each other, start exploring your topic of interest and asking your core questions (University of Mississippi, 2005). For example, "How do you conduct a literature search?" or "What would make you feel empowered to embark on an EBP project?" Wrap up your focus group by giving the group the opportunity to voice any last-minute thoughts or opinions (University of Mississippi, 2005). Ask exit questions such as, "Is there anything else you need to be successful in conducting EBP projects?"

Interviews

A third approach to performing the learning needs assessment is conducting one-on-one interviews with clinical specialists, educators, and unit-based instructors. These individuals work closely with bedside clinicians and can be a valuable resource in identifying the learning needs of staff. They can also provide valuable information about which educational strategies will work best for their respective departments or clinical areas.

ESTABLISH INFRASTRUCTURE

To move an EBP education program forward, the appropriate infrastructure must be available and supported. If an organization provides easy access to EBP resources and creates an expectation of their use, EBP can flourish. Those that do not provide such resources must address this critical need before launching a program.

It is recommended that a healthcare organization be equipped with the following items, at a minimum, to create an environment that is supportive of EBP:

- Access to basic technology, such as computers, Microsoft Office, the internet, etc.
- Access to healthcare databases, such as Medline, PubMed Central, CINAHL, Embase, etc.
- Access to healthcare journals, either online or in print
- Access to health science librarians or informationists

You can access all the above items through an affiliated university or health science library. If your healthcare organization is not affiliated with a university or a health science library, you may consider contacting your local public library or public universities for support. Many public libraries and universities are willing to loan technology, have access to healthcare databases, can assist with acquiring journal articles through interlibrary loans, and employ knowledgeable library personnel. You may also consider using open access databases and journals, which are available to everyone at no charge. To learn more about open access databases and journals, see Chapter 7 in *Johns Hopkins Evidence-Based Practice for Nurses and Healthcare Professionals: Model & Guidelines*, 5th Edition.

IDENTIFY AND DEVELOP MENTORS AND INFORMAL LEADERS

Mentors and informal leaders have an important role in assimilation of EBP into the organizational culture. They provide a safe and supportive environment for staff to move out of their comfort zone as they learn new skills and competencies. You should identify and develop mentors and informal leaders early in creating the EBP education program so that they can serve as advocates for rather than opponents of the program, and model EBP in practice.

Identify and select mentors and informal leaders with care, choosing them from across the organization—different roles, levels, and specialties. Mentors are subject matter experts with the knowledge and skills to move an EBP education program forward, can offer the best support, and have the most at stake to see that EBP is successful. This includes clinical nurse specialists, advance practice providers, and departmental subject matter experts. Informal leaders influence staff at the unit or departmental level. Staff view these people as role models for professional practice, and these people are committed to clinical inquiry and are skillful collaborators and team players. This includes committee chairs, charge nurses, chief residents, etc.

You can develop mentors and informal leaders in many ways. Initially, if the organization has not yet developed experts within their staff, it can find mentors through collaborative opportunities outside of the organization, such as partnerships with schools or consultation with organizations and experts who have developed models. After internal expertise is established, the implementation of an EBP education program throughout the organization results in a self-generating mechanism for developing mentors. For example, members of committees who participate in EBP projects guided by a mentor quickly become mentors to other staff, or staff who participate in EBP fellowships gain the needed skills to lead and consult with staff groups within their home department or throughout the organization.

SELECT TEACHING STRATEGIES

In this section, we discuss a variety of teaching strategies that can be used to teach the foundations of EBP, including both traditional and nontraditional coursework. Any of these strategies can be used to ensure EBP competency. Select the methods that will meet the needs of your organization and are feasible to implement with the resources available to you.

TRADITIONAL COURSEWORK

Traditional coursework is the most effective strategy to learn how to use and apply EBP. It is an instructor-centered approach that includes didactic lectures in combination with activity-based learning. Some traditional coursework options include a fellowship, a workshop, group mentoring, and online modules.

FELLOWSHIP

Overview

The EBP fellowship is geared toward healthcare professionals interested in mastering EBP. Participants will attend an eight-hour class day once a month for 12 months. Class days are comprised of lectures, coaching sessions, and project work. This format is the most time- and resource-intensive option to implement, but it allows for in-depth exposure to EBP content and experts.

> **SPECIAL CONSIDERATIONS**
>
> A fellowship is an excellent way to teach EBP to staff members from different practice settings. However, this approach adds a degree of complexity to identifying an EBP question that is important to the entire class. One strategy for identifying a question is to poll the participants prior to the start of the fellowship to identify a common question or theme that can be used, such as pain management, falls, or pressure ulcer prevention. Another strategy is to identify a common problem across the organization, perhaps alarm management or medication administration, that can be used as an EBP question.

Objectives

The EBP fellowship aims to develop the next generation of EBP champions. After completion of the fellowship, participants will have gained the knowledge, skills, and confidence needed to lead EBP initiatives throughout the organization. Specific objectives include:

1. Describe the evolution of EBP in healthcare, highlighting the role of healthcare professionals.
2. Compare and contrast EBP, quality improvement (QI), and research.
3. Develop a practice question that aligns with organizational priorities.
4. Collaborate with an interprofessional team.
5. Perform a comprehensive and systematic literature search.
6. Critically appraise and synthesize a body of evidence.
7. Establish practice recommendations using the best available scientific and clinical evidence.
8. Develop a plan to implement practice recommendations using implementation science strategies.

9. Collect and analyze data to evaluate the impact of the practice change.
10. Develop a plan to sustain the practice change.
11. Disseminate the results and findings internally, with relevant parties within the organization.
12. Disseminate the results and findings externally, with relevant parties at a professional conference or publication.

Selection Process

Participants are selected for the fellowship through a competitive application and interview process. Sample eligibility criteria include:

1. A minimum of one year of clinical experience
2. A minimum of a bachelor's degree
3. Employed full time by the organization, and must remain employed full time by the organization for the duration of the fellowship
4. Strong written, verbal, and interpersonal skills
5. Demonstrated interest in scholarly work
6. No active discipline

Please note, this is not meant to be an exhaustive list but rather examples of possible eligibility criteria. You may choose to add, remove, or change the criteria based on the composition of your staff.

Sample Timeline

In total, it will take approximately 18 months to implement an EBP fellowship, including the application cycle. For a sample timeline, see Table 3.1.

TABLE 3.1 EBP FELLOWSHIP TIMELINE

DATE	TOPIC
APPLICATION CYCLE	
January	Application opens
January–March	Host information sessions and application support sessions
March	Application closes

April	Interview eligible applicants
May	Select fellows and assign coaches
June	Host meet and greet

CLASSES

July	Class 1: EBP Principles
August	Class 2: EBP Principles
September	Class 3: EBP Principles
October	Class 4: Research Principles
November	Class 5: Research Principles
December	Class 6: Research Principles
January	Class 7: Research Principles
February	Class 8: QI Principles
March	Class 9: Data Principles
April	Class 10: Dissemination Principles
May	Class 11: Dissemination Principles
June	Class 12: Professional Development Principles

ADDITIONAL RESOURCES

An EBP fellowship package is coming soon! It will include sample agendas, slide decks, knowledge checks, activities, and coaching agreements. Keep an eye on our webpage, Hopkins.org/resources, to be the first to know when it is available.

WORKSHOPS

Overview

EBP workshops are geared toward healthcare professionals interested in quickly learning the foundations of EBP. Participants will attend two back-to-back eight-hour class days. Class days are comprised of lectures, activities, and case studies. Didactic content is taught first, followed by an associated hands-on learning opportunity. Workshops are a great opportunity for organizations that want to teach the EBP process in depth but do not have the time or resources to implement a yearlong fellowship. EBP workshops have been successfully implemented in many different settings, including in rural, community, and nonteaching hospitals and large academic medical centers.

Objectives

EBP workshops aim to develop people who are confident and competent to participate in EBP projects and who can one day lead an EBP project. Objectives for EBP workshops are similar to the objectives for the fellowship, but due to time constraints, they do not include implementing the best practice recommendations. Specific objectives include:

1. Describe the evolution of EBP in healthcare, highlighting the role of healthcare professionals.
2. Compare and contrast EBP, QI, and research.
3. Develop a practice question that aligns with organizational priorities.
4. Collaborate with an interprofessional team.
5. Perform a comprehensive and systematic literature search.
6. Critically appraise and synthesize a body of evidence.
7. Establish practice recommendations using the best available scientific and clinical evidence.
8. Identify strategies to implement practice recommendations using implementation science strategies.

Selection Process

There is not an application or interview process to participate in an EBP workshop. One way to recruit participants is to ask organizational leadership—directors, unit managers, committee chairs, etc.—to nominate people who show promise in becoming EBP champions. Another way is to advertise the program throughout the organization and allow people to register for the workshop on a first-come, first-served basis.

Regardless of the method used to recruit participants, you will want to establish eligibility criteria. Similar to the EBP fellowship, sample eligibility criteria include:

1. A minimum of one year of clinical experience
2. A minimum of a bachelor's degree
3. Employed full time by the organization, and must remain employed full time by the organization for the duration of the fellowship
4. Strong written, verbal, and interpersonal skills
5. Demonstrated interest in scholarly work
6. No active discipline

Again, please note, this is not meant to be an exhaustive list but rather examples of possible eligibility criteria. You may choose to add, remove, or change the criteria based on the composition of your staff.

Sample Agenda

In total, it will take about 16 hours to implement an EBP workshop, including opening remarks, breaks, and closing remarks. See Table 3.2 for a sample agenda.

TABLE 3.2 EBP WORKSHOP AGENDA

TIME		TOPIC
DAY 1		
8:00 a.m.	15 min.	Opening remarks
8:15 a.m.	30 min.	Three forms of inquiry
8:45 a.m.	45 min.	Project planning and engagement of relevant parties
9:30 a.m.	45 min.	Finding the root cause of the problem
10:15 a.m.	15 min.	Break
10:30 a.m.	30 min.	Introduction to EBP
11:00 a.m.	75 min.	Writing an EBP question
12:15 p.m.	60 min.	Lunch
1:15 p.m.	90 min.	Searching the literature
2:45 p.m.	15 min.	Break
3:00 p.m.	45 min.	Screening the literature
3:45 p.m.	15 min.	Closing remarks

continues

TABLE 3.2 EBP WORKSHOP AGENDA (CONT.)

TIME		TOPIC
DAY 2		
8:00 a.m.	15 min.	Opening remarks
8:15 a.m.	75 min.	Appraising the literature
9:30 a.m.	15 min.	Break
9:45 a.m.	90 min.	Appraising the literature cont.
11:15 a.m.	45 min.	Summary and synthesis of the literature
12:00 p.m.	60 min.	Lunch
1:00 p.m.	90 min.	Summary and synthesis of the literature cont.
2:30 p.m.	15 min.	Break
2:45 p.m.	60 min.	Translation and implementation of best-practice recommendations
3:45 p.m.	15 min.	Closing remarks

ADDITIONAL RESOURCES

Visit Hopkins.org/resources to download additional resources to support the development of EBP workshops at your organization, such as sample slide decks, knowledge checks, case studies, and activities.

GROUP MENTORING

EBP group mentoring is geared toward healthcare professionals interested in learning the foundations of EBP over time. Participants, typically from the same practice area, are brought together to complete a real-world project with the support of one or two mentors who are experienced in EBP. The group meets regularly for one to two hours at a time to receive didactic content and work on the project. Group mentoring is ideal for practice areas with limited indirect time. Since the sessions are offered in shorter blocks of time, EBP group mentoring can easily fit into a work schedule during lunch hours or regularly scheduled committee meetings.

> **SPECIAL CONSIDERATIONS**
>
> For best results, schedule group mentoring sessions regularly, such as one session per week for 6 to 12 weeks. This also allows enough time for participants to review and digest the content between sessions but not too much time that people start to lose interest in the project.

ONLINE MODULES

Online EBP modules are geared toward healthcare professionals interested in gaining an overview of the EBP process. The modules are brief—containing about three to five hours of content in total— self-paced, and available on demand. The online modules are a great opportunity for organizations that require flexibility in their education program or are seeking new learning opportunities that can be used for orientation, as an adjunct for other training, or for yearly refreshers.

> **ADDITIONAL RESOURCES**
>
> Visit Hopkins.org/resources to purchase online EBP modules. It includes interactive content, instructional videos, and knowledge checks.

NONTRADITIONAL COURSEWORK

Healthcare primarily occurs at the bedside, where traditional coursework is seldom a feasible option. Strategies that incorporate EBP into the fabric of existing processes and structures are most successful in promoting and sustaining a culture of EBP. There are various ways to do this, including committee work, journal clubs, new hire orientation, lunch and learns, and protocol development.

COMMITTEE WORK

Standing professional practice committees, such as standards of care and quality improvement, and their members can use a portion of meeting time to develop an EBP project about a relevant practice issue. Conducting several EBP projects throughout the year as part of the committee's routine work is an excellent way to teach bedside EBP skills and improve practice. Initial projects can be conducted by committee members themselves. As committee members gain more experience in the process, other bedside clinicians can be invited to join future EBP projects to learn the process.

An agenda item devoted to EBP support allows participants to benefit from the collective expertise of the committee while designing and conducting EBP projects in their own departments or units. The committee can also serve as a clearinghouse for communication of EBP projects throughout the organization. Keys to success include dedicating time during the committee meeting to provide updates on EBP projects in progress; developing a standardized method for narrative reporting of EBP projects; providing a template for poster presentations; and developing a web page to post information related to EBP projects, including contact information, so interested individuals can learn more about the projects.

JOURNAL CLUBS

A journal club, which is a wonderful tool to enhance lifelong learning, has great utility for building organizational capacity for EBP. Journal clubs develop skills and build confidence in searching for evidence and using evidence-based information resources, critically appraising evidence, synthesizing evidence, and making recommendations for practical application of findings. Through reading and sharing of ideas, participants work collaboratively to assess a piece of evidence that has direct relevance to their practice. EBP journal club leaders can build on the learning objectives in *Johns Hopkins Evidence-Based Practice for Nurses and Healthcare Professionals: Model & Guidelines,* 5th Edition, to help club members develop essential EBP skills and competencies. Club members can use the tools provided in the appendices of the book as a guide through the EBP process.

Key factors for success include leaders who release club members from patient-care responsibilities during designated meeting times, a club leader well versed in EBP techniques to provide consistent mentorship, and administrative support to procure and distribute evidence. Leaders may also want to explore the use of technology, including online discussion boards and video conferencing recordings, to facilitate an offsite or asynchronous experience that may allow for greater participation.

NEW HIRE ORIENTATION

The bedside, or point of care, provides the perfect venue for capturing teachable moments. Supporting new nursing staff during the first year is often the responsibility of a preceptor or other nurse who has a defined role in unit-based orientation and education of new staff. Preceptor training in EBP principles and concepts can enhance informal, incidental, interpersonal, and interactive learning during the orientation process and throughout the first year of practice. The power of the "how we do things here" mentality is strong. Clinical experiences and interpersonal interactions of the preceptor-learner dyad provide a convenient forum for infusing EBP at the earliest stages of workforce development. The preceptor has the valuable opportunity as a clinical role model to assist the newly hired nurse to think critically, to pose important clinical questions, and to base patient care decisions on evidence. Preceptors with strong EBP skills make it clear that EBP is part of the nursing culture. Key factors for success include training preceptors to model expected EBP behaviors and skills and taking advantage of each teaching encounter to impart the importance of seeking out and translating evidence to patient care.

LUNCH AND LEARNS

Monthly lunch-and-learn sessions are also becoming increasingly popular to reinforce continuing education because they do not require nurse leaders to release staff from patient care responsibilities. Scheduled during staggered lunch periods, these sessions can reinforce content over time and provide targeted learning-application activities to be completed between sessions.

PROTOCOL DEVELOPMENT

Most organizations have a defined process for protocol or policy development, review, and revision. These activities present first-rate opportunities to build organizational capacity for EBP by cultivating EBP skills and competencies in the teams that develop, review, and revise clinical practice standards. *Johns Hopkins Evidence-Based Practice for Nurses and Healthcare Professionals: Model & Guidelines,* 5th Edition, can walk teams through the EBP process step by step to support protocol development. Keys for success include making sure that clinical questions are important to the content of the protocol; assigning an EBP mentor or fellow as a consistent resource to the protocol development and review team; and communicating the results of the EBP review, along with education surrounding new or revised protocols.

EVALUATE THE PROGRAM

Once your EBP education program has launched, you will want to evaluate the program to ensure that the program is meeting your participants' needs. After each educational activity, gather staff feedback using an evaluation questionnaire. Listen to your staff! Be responsive to their comments, questions, and concerns, and make alterations to the education plan, if needed, to ensure its effectiveness over time.

> **ADDITIONAL RESOURCES**
>
> Visit Hopkins.org/resources to download additional resources to evaluate the EBP education program at your organization, including a sample evaluation questionnaire.

CONCLUSION

Infusing EBP knowledge and skills throughout a healthcare organization involves a comprehensive educational plan that employs multiple educational strategies, based on the needs of staff and organizational resources. The key to the plan's effectiveness rests not only with the education provided and the teaching approaches used but also with the organization's ability to build capacity through development and support of mentors, both at central and departmental levels. Mentors are instrumental in helping the organization build a culture of continual learning that encourages staff to question clinical practice and promotes EBP to examine practice issues. Using a steering committee to develop and frequently evaluate the comprehensive plan can also help ensure that adequate resources are devoted to EBP training and that necessary alterations are made to the educational plan to ensure its effectiveness over time.

PART 4
WORKBOOK LEARNING ACTIVITIES AND ANSWER KEY

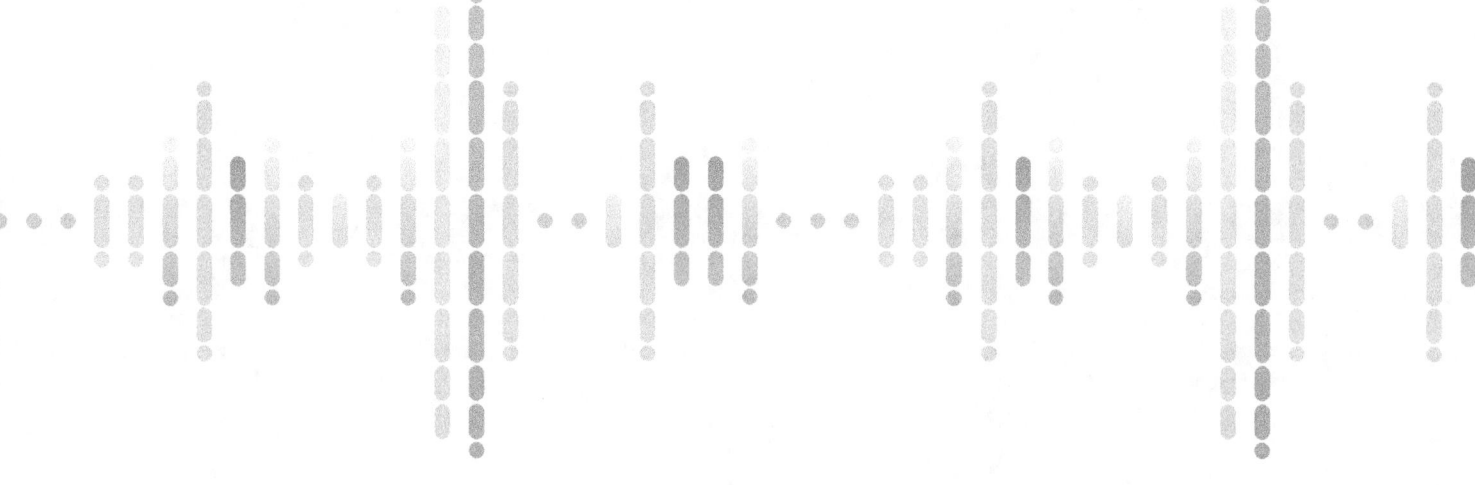

The sections in this part correspond chapter by chapter to the *Workbook for Johns Hopkins Evidence-Based Practice for Nurses and Healthcare Professionals,* Fifth Edition.

The figure numbers here correspond to the workbook and do not correspond with the numbering system in other parts of this guide.

1

EVIDENCE-BASED PRACTICE: PAST, PRESENT, AND FUTURE

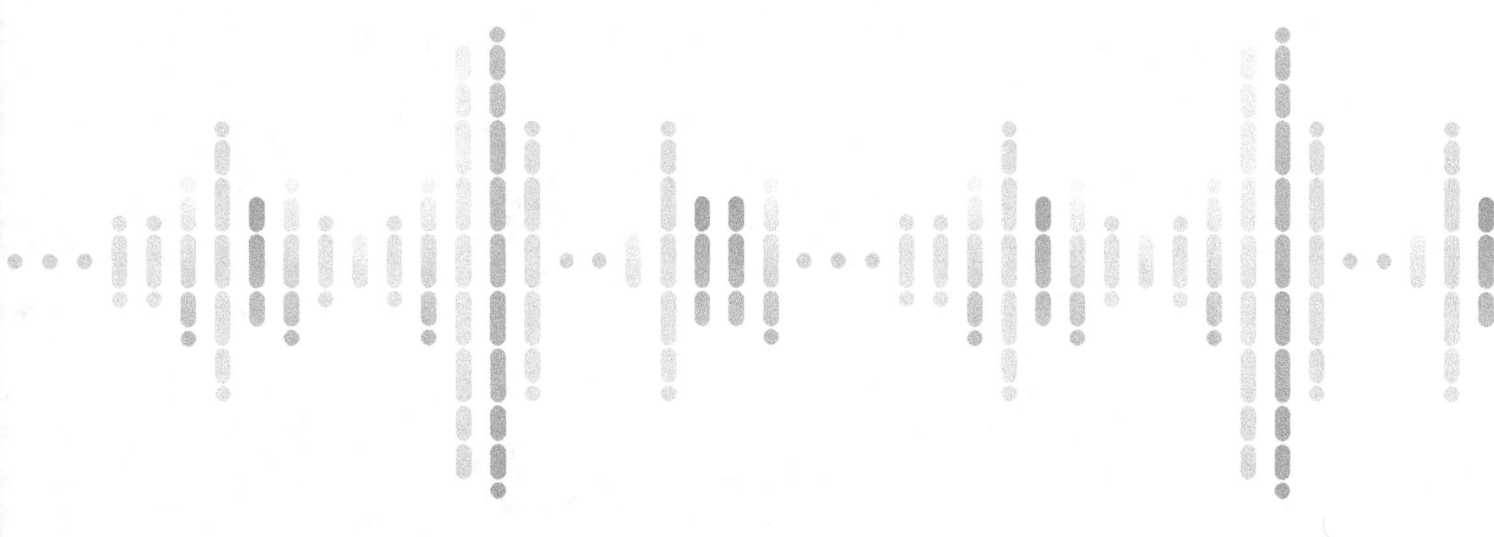

LEARNING OBJECTIVES

- 1.1 Compare and contrast practice based on evidence and one based on tradition (analyzing)

- 1.2 Describe three ways artificial intelligence (AI) may promote EBP (understanding)

- 1.3 Demonstrate how EBP can be used to address health equity on a local level (applying)

LEARNING ACTIVITIES

Before completion of the learning activities, learners are directed to do the following:

- Read Chapter 1
- Read the article at https://nursingaura.com/44-difference-between-evidence-based-practice-and-traditional-nursing/

Learning Activity 1.1

Create a table differentiating evidence-based and tradition-based practices.

CHARACTERISTICS	EBP	TRADITION
DEFINITION	A decision-making process that integrates the best available research evidence, clinical expertise, and patient preferences.	Practices and interventions that are based on historical, cultural, or familial traditions, often passed down through generations.
SOURCES OF KNOWLEDGE	Empirical research, scientific studies, and systematic reviews.	Cultural knowledge, historical practices, oral traditions, and long-established methods.
FLEXIBILITY	Adaptable to new research findings and evolving evidence.	Often rigid, based on longstanding customs or cultural beliefs.
APPROACH TO CHANGE	Embraces changes when new evidence contradicts current practices.	Resistant to change, as practices are deeply rooted in tradition.

Learning Activity 1.2

Identify and describe three ways AI may promote EBP.

Answer: There may be several correct answers to this question. Some include: speed up evidence integration, assist with analyzing large volumes of data, provide living systematic reviews, and make the EBP process easier.

Learning Activity 1.3

After reading excerpt 1 from the case study, outline steps the team should take or consider to address health equity through the EBP process.

Answer: There are several ways to answer the question correctly. Some include:

1. Build a diverse EBP team, including people with a variety of backgrounds, experiences, and perspectives.
2. Understand that hospital falls impact older adults and people with comorbidities more than other groups.
3. Understand that some groups of people will not seek medical care or will seek medical care too late. This includes people that cannot afford the high cost of healthcare, people that are uninsured or underinsured, and people that fear the healthcare system. These groups of people may be underrepresented in the literature.
4. Understand that different healthcare facilities have access to different resources. Some facilities may not have the resources needed to implement large-scale, expensive initiatives. Be sure to develop recommendations that are inclusive of all backgrounds.

DISCUSSION QUESTIONS

1. What are the primary barriers to implementing EBP in clinical settings, and how might healthcare organizations work to overcome these obstacles?
2. How did the COVID-19 pandemic underscore the importance of EBP for clinicians, particularly in terms of quickly accessing and evaluating available evidence? What lessons can be learned for future healthcare challenges?
3. In what ways could emerging technologies, like AI, change the landscape of EBP? What role should clinicians play in ensuring the reliability and accuracy of AI-generated evidence?
4. How can EBP be leveraged to address healthcare inequalities? What strategies could be implemented to ensure that EBP considerations start at the local level and address diverse community needs?
5. Despite advancements in EBP, some healthcare providers continue to rely on traditional practices. What factors contribute to this reliance, and how can a culture of critical thinking and continuous learning be fostered to encourage wider adoption of EBP?

THE JOHNS HOPKINS EVIDENCE-BASED PRACTICE (JHEBP) MODEL FOR NURSES AND HEALTHCARE PROFESSIONALS (HCPs) PROCESS OVERVIEW

LEARNING OBJECTIVES

- 2.1 Differentiate between quality improvement, EBP, and research (analyzing)

- 2.2 Describe the JHEBP model and PET process (understanding)

- 2.3 Demonstrate knowledge of the appropriate steps in the PET process (applying)

LEARNING ACTIVITIES

Before completion of the learning activity, learners are directed to do the following:

- Read Chapter 2
- Listen to this podcast: https://podcasts.apple.com/us/podcast/ep-4-johns-hopkins-nursing-center-for-nursing-inquiry/id1478145611?i=1000448670863
- Download the EBP Project Steps and Overview (Appendix A) and the Gantt chart from Hopkins.org/resources

Learning Activity 2.1

Part 1: In your own words, define the following:

Quality improvement	Improves systems and processes on a local level; may use a model such as PDSA or Lean Sigma
Research	Generates new knowledge; uses a structured approach/scientific method
Evidence-based practice	Uses existing evidence to determine best practices

Part 2: Given the following statements, select the appropriate category (QI, research, or EBP).

___QI____ The nurses in Labor and Delivery at XYZ Hospital want to improve the time it takes for new mothers to be evaluated by the lactation nurse.

_Research _ A group from ABC University wants to better understand the impact of social media on children born to single parents.

___EBP____ The Nursing Department at XYZ Hospital wants to ensure they provide the best support for families of children recently diagnosed with leukemia.

Learning Activity 2.2

Describe what sparks an EBP project. Once initiated, what are the three phases the team will move through? What happens in each of these phases?

Answer: Inquiry sparks an EBP project. The three phases are the PET process: Practice Question, Evidence, and Translation. In the practice question phase, the team explores and defines the problem to develop an EBP question. In the evidence phase, the team searches for, screens, and appraises evidence to develop best-evidence recommendations.

Learning Activity 2.3

Order the 16 steps of the JHEBP model by placing the correct numbers in front of each step.

14	Create an implementation/action plan	3	Write the EBP question
11	Assess the risk, fit, feasibility, and acceptability of best-evidence recommendations	7	Summarize the evidence
5	Conduct targeted search or exhaustive search and screening	4	Conduct best-evidence search and appraisal
10	Record best-evidence recommendations	12	Identify practice-setting specific recommendations
8	Organize the data	15	Implement
1	Explore and describe the problem	16	Monitor sustainability and identify next steps
6	Appraise the evidence	9	Synthesize the findings
13	Identify an implementation framework	2	Develop the problem statement

DISCUSSION QUESTIONS

1. What are the key components of the revised JHEBP model, and how does this updated framework improve upon previous versions in supporting effective EBP?

2. The PET process consists of 16 steps. How can healthcare organizations ensure that healthcare professionals are adequately trained and supported at each step of the process to successfully implement EBP?

3. How can coaching and mentorship contribute to the success of EBP initiatives? What strategies could be employed to foster these relationships within healthcare teams?

4. What role does organizational commitment play in the successful adoption of the PET process? How can leaders at various levels promote a culture that values EBP?

5. Healthcare professionals come from diverse educational backgrounds and levels of experience. What are some ways that organizations can tailor EBP training to accommodate this diversity, ensuring that all staff are equipped to utilize the PET process effectively?

3

PRACTICE QUESTION PHASE: THE PROBLEM

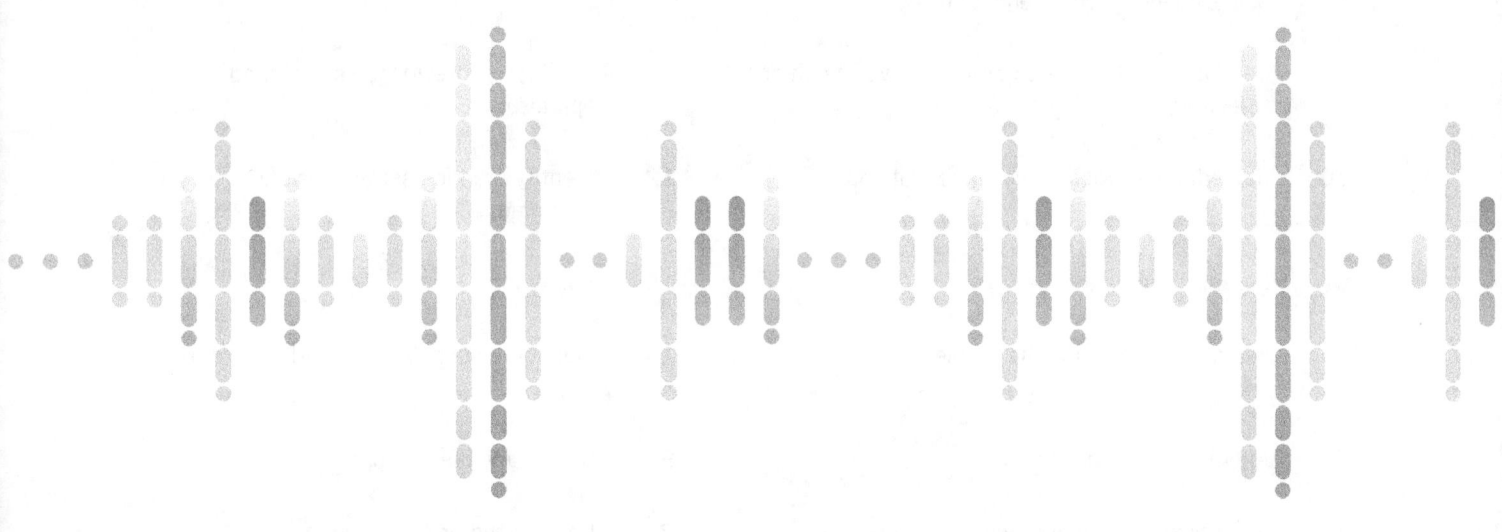

LEARNING OBJECTIVES

- 3.1 Identify strategies used to define problems (understanding)
- 3.2 Differentiate between problems, solutions, and symptoms (analyzing)
- 3.3 Construct a problem statement (creating)

LEARNING ACTIVITIES

Before completion of the learning activity, learners are directed to do the following:

- Read Chapter 3
- Read this article: https://online.hbs.edu/blog/post/root-cause-analysis
- Review the Question Development Tool (Appendix B)
- Download the Fishbone diagram from the resources page (Hopkins.org/resources)

Learning Activity 3.1

Draw a line to match each strategy with the corresponding rationale.

STRATEGY	RATIONALE
Examine the problem critically without making assumptions to ensure the final statement defines the specific problem.	Gives the team time to gather information, observe, listen, and probe to ensure a true understanding of the problem
Challenge assumptions.	Helps the team avoid conjecture and question everyday processes and practices that are taken for granted
Ask clarifying questions.	Helps the team get to the specific problem by using question words such as when, what, how
State the problem differently.	Helps gain clarity by using different verbs
Expand and contract the problem.	Helps the team understand whether the problem is part of a larger problem or is made up of many smaller problems
Refrain from blaming the problem on external forces or focusing attention on the wrong aspect of the problem.	Keeps the team focused on processes and systems as the team moves to define the EBP question
Describe in precise terms the perceived gap between what one sees and what one wants to see.	Allows the team to assess the current state and envision a future state in which broken components are fixed, risks are prevented, new evidence is accepted, and missing elements are provided

Learning Activity 3.2

Identify whether the following statements describe the symptom(s) of a problem, a problem, or a solution to a problem.

1. Central venous catheters (CVC) are necessary tools to care for critically ill patients. However, improper insertion, maintenance, and removal of central lines can lead to bacterial and fungal infections.

    a. Symptoms of a problem

    b. Problem

    c. Solution to a problem

    Answer: b

2. There is an increase in central line–associated bloodstream infections (CLABSIs) in the Department of Surgery at a large, academic medical center. CLABSIs can lead to increased length of stay, healthcare costs, and morbidity and mortality.

    a. Symptoms of a problem

    b. Problem

    c. Solution to a problem

    Answer: a

3. Using an equipment bundle when inserting a central line can help reduce CLABSIs. A central line equipment bundle includes and organizes all the equipment needed to prepare, insert, secure, and dress a CVC.

    a. Symptoms of a problem

    b. Problem

    c. Solution to a problem

    Answer: c

Learning Activity 3.3

Complete the problems portion of the Question Development Tool (Appendix B; see Figure 3.1) using the case study excerpt from Chapter 1 of the workbook.

Question Development Tool

Purpose: This form guides the EBP team in developing an answerable EBP question. It is meant to be fluid and dynamic as the team engages in the question development process. As the team becomes familiar with the evidence base for the topic of interest, they revisit, revise, and refine the question, search terms, search strategy, and sources of evidence.

If viewing this online, hover over bold text for more information

What is the local problem? *(the response can be a bulleted list or phrases)*
Over the past quarter, there has been a 35% increase in falls on your unit. The falls on your unit were caused by a variety of issues, but most commonly because of patient-related factors (e.g. age, medical conditions, medications, etc.) or environmental factors (e.g. such as clutter, wet floors, poor lighting, etc.).
Why is this problem important and relevant? What would happen if it was not addressed?
The problem is important and relevant because hospital falls can lead to increased length of stay, health care costs, and morbidity and mortality.
What is the current practice in the EBP team's setting?
To prevent patient falls, your organization currently employs a scored screening tool to assess fall risk, environmental safety checks, patient and family education, and, when needed, wristband identification, position alarms, and sitters.
What data from the EBP team's setting indicates there is a problem?
• *Fall rates* • *Chart audits*
Considering all of the information above, create a concise problem statement below.
Patient falls during a hospital stay are a significant concern because they can increase length of stay, health care costs, and morbidity and mortality. Fall rates on your unit are on the rise despite adherence to hospital-wide fall prevention practices. You need to better understand best practices for fall prevention in hospitalized adults.
Will this be a broad or intervention EBP question?
☒ Broad ☐ Intervention

FIGURE 3.1 Question Development Tool (Appendix B, part 1), answer key.

DISCUSSION QUESTIONS

1. Why is it essential to accurately define the practice problem before formulating an EBP question, and what are the potential consequences of failing to do so?

2. What techniques or tools (e.g., root cause analysis, data exploration) are most effective in narrowing down and defining the practice problem? How can these methods enhance the quality of the EBP process?

3. How can interprofessional collaboration contribute to a more comprehensive understanding of the practice problem? What benefits does an interprofessional approach bring to this phase of the PET process?

4. What elements should a well-developed problem statement include to ensure it is compelling and actionable for the intended audience? How can a sense of urgency in a problem statement influence decision-making and support for EBP initiatives?

5. Reflect on a practice problem within your field or experience. What steps would you take to refine this problem into a clear, concise statement that could guide an EBP question?

PRACTICE QUESTION PHASE: THE EBP QUESTION

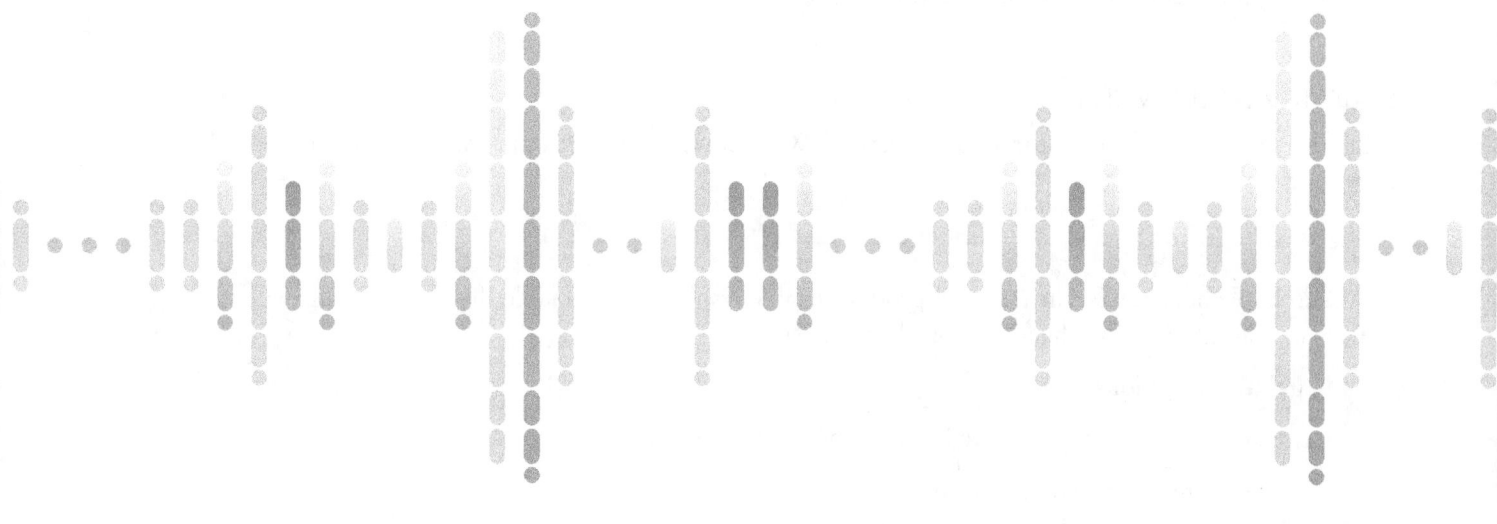

LEARNING OBJECTIVES

- 4.1 Describe a searchable question (understanding)
- 4.2 Differentiate between broad and intervention questions (analyzing)
- 4.3 Construct two types of EBP questions (creating)

LEARNING ACTIVITIES

Before completion of the learning activities, learners are directed to do the following:

- Read Chapter 4
- Listen to the following podcast: https://podcasts.apple.com/us/podcast/ep-9-johns-hopkins-nursing-center-for-nursing-inquiry/id1478145611?i=1000448670860
- Review the Question Development Tool (Appendix B)

Learning Activity 4.1

What does it mean to have a searchable question? What components are important in creating a searchable question?

> A searchable question is one that will produce usable results. It will enable the team to find evidence. Learners should identify the following characteristics:
>
> Searchable questions...
>
> - Are concise and focused to facilitate a more efficient search
> - May be limited to two to three main concepts
> - Often address who, what, when, where, why, and how of the problem or issue at hand
> - Can be created with question frameworks
> - Are neither too broad or vague nor too specific

Learning Activity 4.2

Complete the following table, differentiating between broad and intervention questions.

	DEFINITION	PURPOSE	SEARCH YIELD	COMPONENTS
Broad	Type of question that looks for all available evidence on the topic	Broad EBP questions are a good place to start when the interprofessional team lacks extensive knowledge of the topic at hand.	Wide variety, lots of evidence	Topic, population, and place
Intervention	Type of question that provides more precise knowledge to inform decisions or actions	Intervention EBP questions are generally informed by evidence or experience, often comparing two or more interventions.	Specific and more limited body of evidence	Population Setting outcome

Learning Activity 4.3

Part 1: Identify the relevant elements of the EBP question in the following scenario:

Central venous catheters (CVC) are necessary tools to care for critically ill children in the Pediatric Intensive Care Unit (PICU). However, improper insertion, maintenance, and removal of central lines can lead to bacterial and fungal infections, known as central line–associated bloodstream infections (CLABSIs). CLABSIs can lead to increased length of stay, healthcare costs, and morbidity and mortality.

Population:	Children
Setting:	PICU
Topic (for broad questions) or Interventions (for intervention questions):	CLABSIs
Outcomes (as needed):	N/A

Part 2: Now, identify the relevant elements of the EBP question in the following scenario (new information is underlined):

Central venous catheters (CVC) are necessary tools to care for critically ill children in the Pediatric Intensive Care Unit (PICU). However, improper insertion, maintenance, and removal of central lines can lead to bacterial and fungal infections, known as central line–associated bloodstream infections (CLABSIs). CLABSIs can lead to increased length of stay, healthcare costs, and morbidity and mortality. <u>Using an equipment bundle when inserting a central line is a widespread practice to help reduce CLABSIs.</u>

Population:	Children
Setting:	PICU
Topic (for broad questions) or Interventions (for intervention questions):	Equipment bundle
Outcomes (as needed):	CLABSI rates

Part 3: Using the relevant elements identified above, craft a *broad* EBP question and an *intervention* EBP question.

Broad:

In/among (population and/or setting), what are the best practices/strategies/interventions for/regarding (topic)?

> Among children in the PICU, what are the best practices regarding CLABSIs?

Intervention:

According to the evidence, in/among (population and/or setting), what is the impact of (intervention) on (outcome)?

> According to the evidence, among children in the PICU, what is the impact of bundled equipment on CLABSI rates?

Learning Activity 4.4

After reading the case study excerpts in Chapter 4 of the workbook, complete the remaining sections of the Question Development Tool (Appendix B; see Figure 4.1). For this case study, only develop a *broad* question.

Question Development Tool

Purpose: This form guides the EBP team in developing an answerable EBP question. It is meant to be fluid and dynamic as the team engages in the question development process. As the team becomes familiar with the evidence base for the topic of interest, they revisit, revise, and refine the question, search terms, search strategy, and sources of evidence.

If viewing this online, hover over bold text for more information

What is the local problem? *(the response can be a bulleted list or phrases)*

Over the past quarter, there has been a 35% increase in falls on your unit. The falls on your unit were caused by a variety of issues, but most commonly because of patient-related factors (e.g. age, medical conditions, medications, etc.) or environmental factors (e.g. such as clutter, wet floors, poor lighting, etc.).

Why is this problem important and relevant? What would happen if it was not addressed?

The problem is important and relevant because hospital falls can lead to increased length of stay, health care costs, and morbidity and mortality.

What is the current practice in the EBP team's setting?

To prevent patient falls, your organization currently employs a scored screening tool to assess fall risk, environmental safety checks, patient and family education, and, when needed, wristband identification, position alarms, and sitters.

What data from the EBP team's setting indicates there is a problem?

- *Fall rates*
- *Chart audits*

Considering all of the information above, create a concise problem statement below.

Patient falls during a hospital stay are a significant concern because they can increase length of stay, health care costs, and morbidity and mortality. Fall rates on your unit are on the rise despite adherence to hospital-wide fall prevention practices. You need to better understand best practices for fall prevention in hospitalized adults.

Will this be a broad or intervention EBP question?

☒ Broad   ☐ Intervention

FIGURE 4.1 Question Development Tool (Appendix B), annotated.

continues

Identify the relevant elements of the EBP question *(some items may not be used)*	
Population	Adults
Setting	Hospital, in-patient
Topic (for broad questions) or **Intervention**(s) (for intervention questions)	Fall prevention
Outcomes (as needed)	N/A

Use the information above, and the sentence templates below, to construct the EBP question.

For Broad EBP Questions:

In/among _**adults in the hospital**_ , what are ⟨best practices/strategies/interventions⟩ for/regarding
        (population and/or setting)

**fall prevention** ?
  (topic)

For Intervention EBP Questions:

According to the evidence, in/among _____ , what is the impact of _____ on _____?
                          (population and/or setting)   *(intervention*)*   *(outcome)*

*if comparing more than one intervention, provide the interventions and separate them with the phrase "as compared to"

Record the completed EBP question below.

In hospitalized adults, what are the best practices for fall prevention?

If needed after a preliminary evidence search/review, record an updated or revised EBP question here.

> Note: In general, teams should avoid directional terms such as "reduce" or "increase" which may bias the results of the search. For this example, the word "prevention" was used to represent interventions and to narrow the search from the all-encompassing term "falls."

FIGURE 4.1 Question Development Tool (Appendix B), annotated (cont.).

5

THE INTERPROFESSIONAL TEAM

LEARNING OBJECTIVES

- 5.1 Identify impacted parties (understanding)
- 5.2 Review communication plan resource (understanding)

LEARNING ACTIVITIES

Before completion of the learning activities, learners are directed to do the following:

- Read Chapter 5
- Listen to the following podcast: https://podcasts.hopkinsmedicine.org/episode-50-engaging-staff-in-inquiry-work/
- Review the Impacted Groups Analysis and Communication Resource (Hopkins.com/resources)

Learning Activity 5.1

Identify the four roles impacted groups may fill and define.

Answers:

1. Responsible: completes identified tasks, has recommending authority
2. Consultant: provides input (subject matter expertise), no decision-making authority
3. Informant: Notified of progress and changes, no input on decisions
4. Approval: Signs off on recommendations, may veto

Learning Activity 5.2

After reading the excerpt from the case study in Chapter 5 of the workbook, complete the highlighted portion of the Impacted Groups Analysis and Communication Resource (see Figure 5.1). Recall roles may be filled by more than one individual or group.

Impacted Group Analysis and Communication Resource

Impacted groups analysis matrix:							(Adapted from http://www.tools4dev.org/)
Impacted Individual/ Group Name and Title:	Role: (select all that apply) Responsibility, Approval, Consult, Inform	Impact Level: How much does the project impact them? (minor, moderate, significant)	Influence Level: How much influence do they have over the project? (minor, moderate, significant)	What matters most to the individual or group?	How could the individual or group contribute to the project?	How could the individul/group impede the project?	Strategy(s) for engaging the individual/ group:
Sofia - Clinical Nurse Specialist	Responsible Sofia will likely be a member of the core EBP team and actively involved in the day-to-day activities of the project. As a clinical nurse specialist and staunch advocate for patient safety, she has in-depth knowledge of the problem, and, since she is valued for her clinical experience and expertise, will likely serve as a change agent when the time comes to implement interventions.	Significant	Significant				
Ravi - Vendor	Inform Since Ravi is a third-party vendor, he has no input on unit-based decisions. However, depending on your intervention, he would likely need to be informed of changes to the supply order. For example, if your unit decides to implement fall prevention signs in each room, you may need to order more	Minor	Minor				

© 2025 The Johns Hopkins Hospital/Johns Hopkins University School of Nursing

Keep in mind, you may assess impact and influence differently for the given scenario.

FIGURE 5.1 Impacted Groups Analysis and Communication Resource answer key.

DISCUSSION QUESTIONS

1. What are the essential qualities or skills that EBP team leaders should possess to effectively lead an interprofessional team? How can these qualities contribute to the team's overall success?

2. In what ways can diverse healthcare professionals contribute unique perspectives to an EBP project? What are some strategies to ensure that all voices and specialties are heard and valued within the team?

3. How can EBP teams identify and involve relevant stakeholders outside of the core team? What benefits do these stakeholders bring to the EBP process, and how can their involvement enhance project outcomes?

4. What are some common challenges interprofessional EBP teams may face, and what strategies can be employed to overcome these obstacles to maintain effective teamwork and engagement?

5. How can interprofessional EBP teams establish and maintain accountability throughout the project? What tools or methods might help sustain team motivation and commitment to the project's goals?

6
EVIDENCE PHASE: INTRODUCTION TO EVIDENCE

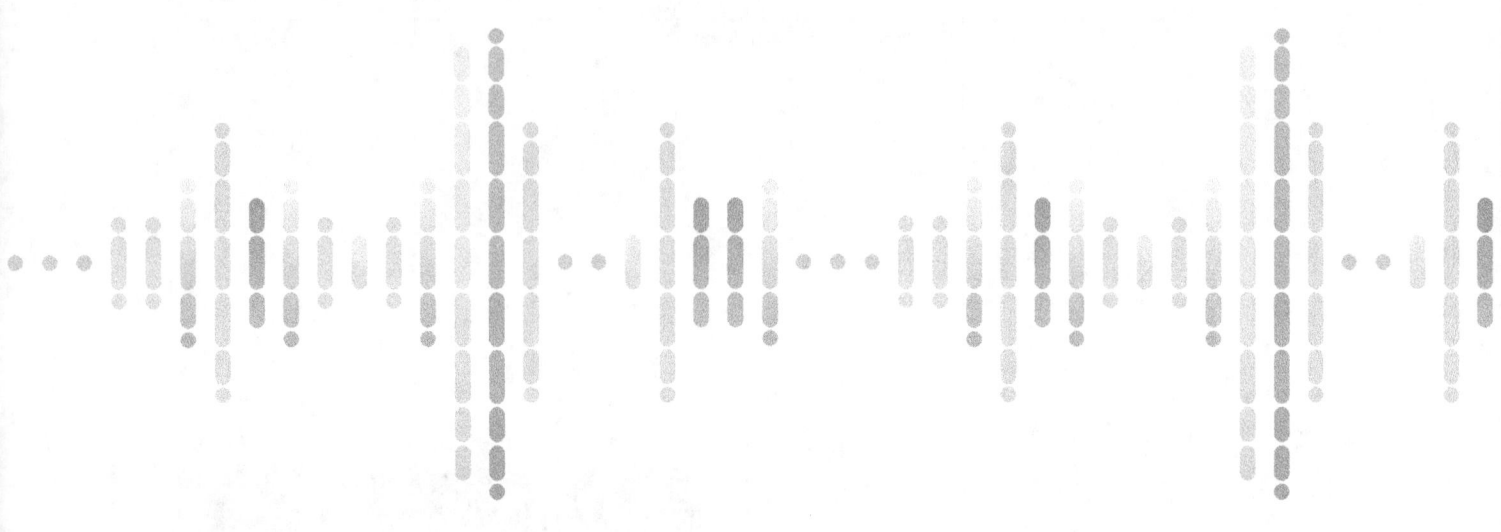

LEARNING OBJECTIVES

- 6.1 Differentiate between the main types of evidence (analyzing)
- 6.2 Describe support for decision-making (understanding)
- 6.3 Select appropriate approaches to generate evidence (evaluating)

LEARNING ACTIVITIES

Before completion of the learning activities, learners are directed to do the following:

- Read Chapter 6
- Listen to the following podcast: https://podcasts.apple.com/us/podcast/ep20-johns-hopkins-center-for-nursing-inquiry-different/id1478145611?i=1000480879172
- Download the Evidence Terminology and Considerations Guide (Appendix F) (Hopkins.org/tools)

Learning Activity 6.1

Align the descriptions with the appropriate type of evidence. Write the letters of the corresponding descriptions in the appropriate boxes.

a. Uses systematic inquiry to answer questions or solve problems

b. Allows clinicians to rely on the expertise of content and research methods experts to process literature and generate recommendations

c. Categorized by the design, not the intent

d. Serves as independent support for decision-making in healthcare

e. Published information that was not generated from a research study but rather from personal, professional, or clinical experience

f. Examples include clinical practice guidelines, literature reviews with a systematic approach, and evidence summaries

g. Types include expert opinion, case report, programmatic experience, and literature review without a systematic approach

h. Studies that have undergone a methodical process for collection and critical evaluation

i. Can be categorized by both the methodologic approach (quantitative, qualitative, or mixed-methods) and the design

j. Provides low support for decision-making

k. Scientific data in the form of qualitative and quantitative data

l. Also known as filtered or secondary literature

PRE-APPRAISED EVIDENCE
b, d, f, h, l

SINGLE STUDIES
a, c, i, k

ANECDOTAL EVIDENCE
e, g, j

Learning Activity 6.2

Part 1: Describe support for decision-making.

Answer: Support for decision-making is a way of categorizing the evidence that is based on the type of evidence and the details of the approach (design) the authors used to generate their findings and conclusions.

Part 2: Identify the degree of support for decision-making provided by these examples.

Pre-appraised evidence	Independent
Single studies with formal study designs	Strong or moderate
Anecdotal evidence	Low

Learning Activity 6.3

Select appropriate approaches to generate evidence.

1. Researchers are trying to gain an in-depth understanding of online gaming addiction in adolescents, including opinions, meanings, and motivations. Little has been explored on this topic, so they hope to generate some hypotheses and directions for further study. The researchers would be best served to conduct:

    a. A quantitative study to understand the scope of the problem in actual numbers

    b. A qualitative study to thoroughly explore the issue and bring meaning to a fairly new phenomenon

    c. A mixed-methods study to explore the phenomenon from all aspects and focus on more specific pieces of the problem

    Answer: b

2. A research team has developed a new device to prevent pressure injuries in hospitalized adults. They need to determine how effective this device is in preventing injury. They need to conduct:

    a. A qualitative study to understand how patients feel about the device and learn about their experiences with pressure injuries

    b. A mixed-methods study to both measure the effectiveness of the device and understand nurses' thoughts on pressure injury prevention

    c. A quantitative study to generate numerical data reflecting the effectiveness of the device

    Answer: c

3. Researchers would like to determine if a structured RN-to-RN handoff works to convey important patient care issues and identify any barriers that may exist to prevent its full-scale adoption. They should conduct:

   a. A mixed-methods study using a quantitative measure of the number of patient care issues conveyed and interviews with staff to understand any barriers to providing this type of handoff

   b. A qualitative study to define handoff and explore potential barriers experienced by nurses

   c. A quantitative study looking at the number of patient care issues conveyed through the handoff process

   Answer: a

DISCUSSION QUESTIONS

1. How does the Johns Hopkins EBP model define "evidence" within the context of EBP, and why is it important for EBP teams to clearly understand this definition?

2. What are the key types of evidence that an EBP team might encounter, and how can each type contribute uniquely to addressing a practice question?

3. What recent changes to the Johns Hopkins EBP model influence how evidence is assessed, and how do these changes reflect advancements in evidence-based healthcare?

4. Why is it crucial for EBP teams to align their assessment methods with contemporary standards and practices in healthcare, and what impact might this alignment have on patient care outcomes?

5. During the literature search, what methods can EBP teams employ to efficiently screen and appraise different types of evidence? How do these methods ensure the selection of high-quality, relevant evidence?

7

EVIDENCE PHASE: THE EVIDENCE SEARCH AND SCREENING

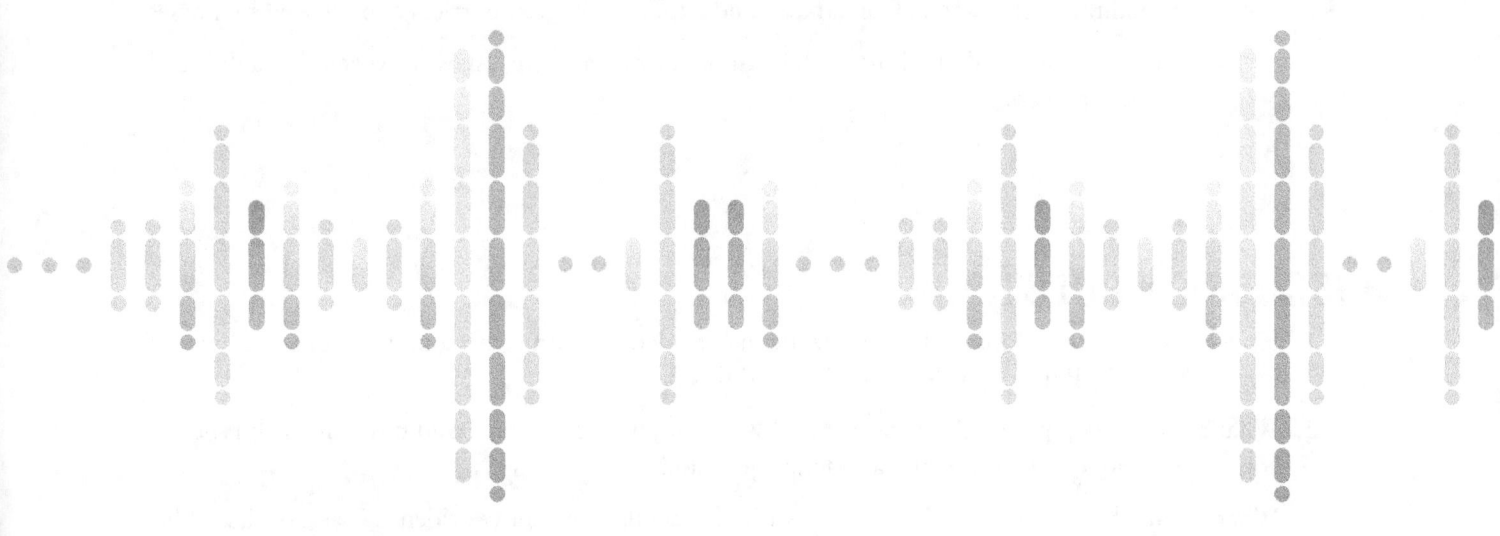

LEARNING OBJECTIVES

- 7.1 Differentiate between a best-evidence search and an exhaustive search (analyzing)
- 7.2 Develop a replicable search string (applying)
- 7.3 Identify ways to screen evidence (understanding)

LEARNING ACTIVITIES

Before completion of the learning activities, learners are directed to do the following:

- Read Chapter 7
- Listen to the following podcast: https://podcasts.apple.com/us/podcast/episode-55-searching-pre-appraised-evidence-part-1/id1478145611?i=1000658675607
- Listen to the following podcast: https://podcasts.apple.com/us/podcast/episode-56-who-produces-sources-of-pre-appraised/id1478145611?i=1000658675608
- Listen to the following podcast: https://podcasts.apple.com/us/podcast/episode-57-repositories-of-pre-appraised-evidence/id1478145611?i=1000658675782
- Download the Searching and Screening Tool (Appendix C) (Hopkins.org/tools)

Learning Activity 7.1

Part 1: Differentiate between a best-evidence search and an exhaustive search.

TYPE OF SEARCH	DEFINITION	BEST USE
Best-evidence	Focused process to identify key foundational articles and existing syntheses (pre-appraised evidence), but not all articles on a topic	Time-sensitive decision-making, guiding internal decisions, informing larger research projects; as the first search of the EBP project
Exhaustive	Systematically identifies all relevant literature with structured, comprehensive, and reproducible methods	Inform clinical questions or practice

Part 2: Name three sources of best evidence.

Answer: There are several original sources of pre-appraised evidence. These include Cochrane Library, JBI (Joanna Briggs Institute), the National Institute for Health and Care Excellence (NICE), US Preventative Services Taskforce (USPSTF), AHRQ Evidence-based Practice Center (EPC) reports, and World Health Organization (WHO) guidelines.

Clinical practice guidelines from professional organizations can be found at ECRI Guidelines Trust, Guideline Central, Physiotherapy Evidence Database (PEDro), and Trip Database.

Learning Activity 7.2

Part 1: Reflect back on the key elements you identified in the Question Development Tool (Apprendix B). Using those elements, fill out Appendix C, Searching and Screening Tool (see Figure 7.1).

Section I: Key Elements of the EBP Question	
Identify the key elements of the EBP question (*from the Question Development Tool*)	
Population	**Adults**
Setting	**Hospital, in-patient**
Topic or Intervention(s)	**Fall prevention**
Outcomes (as needed)	

FIGURE 7.1 Searching and Screening Tool (Appendix C, Section I), answer key.

> **Facilitator Note:** Answers and results for the above search questions may differ depending on a number of factors including search terms used, databases searched, and limitations used.

Part 2: Conduct a best-evidence search (see Figure 7.2) using these key elements and one of the sources identified in Learning Activity 7.1, part 2. Were you able to find a clinical practice guideline, literature review with a systematic approach, or evidence summary? If so, you could appraise the evidence and move to a targeted search. However, for this exercise we will move to an exhaustive search (see Figure 7.3).

Section II: Best-Evidence Search
Does pre-appraised evidence exist in the form of clinical practice guidelines (CPGs), literature reviews with a systematic approach (LRSAs) or evidence summaries?

☐ Yes → Appraise using the Pre-Appraised Evidence Appraisal Tool (Appendix E1)
   o Is the evidence suitable and adequate quality?
      ☐ Yes → Complete targeted search for additional evidence based on search date in pre-appraised evidence to determine if relevant evidence has been published in the interim
      ☐ No → Skip to Section III (exhaustive search)
 	
☒ No → Skip to Section III (Exhaustive Search)

FIGURE 7.2 Searching and Screening Tool (Appendix C), Section II.

Part 3: Complete the provided sections of the Searching and Screening Tool (Appendix C).

Section III: Exhaustive Search and Screening	
Complete the table below using the population, setting, topic or intervention(s) and outcomes identified in Section I. List the element and associated terms to build a full search concept.	
EBP Question Element	Possible Search Terms (*synonyms, alternative spellings or brand names*)
1) Adult	Adult, aged 18 and over
2) Hospital, in-patient	Hospital*, admitted, inpatient, patient, ward
3) Fall prevention	Fall prevent*, fall interventions, accidental falls/prevention and control,

FIGURE 7.3 Searching and Screening Tool (Appendix C), Section III, answer key.

Part 4: Using the information you gathered above, spend some time developing a replicable search string for at least one database. Conduct the search and record the number of articles you found (see Figure 7.4).

What databases will you search?	
X CINAHL X MEDLINE (PubMed) X Embase	☐ PsychINFO ☐ Epistemonikos ☐ Other:
What are the inclusion and exclusion criteria?	
Inclusion: adult, inpatient, English language, fall prevention,	Exclusion: non-hospital, pediatrics,
What date limit will you use and why?	
5 years because we anticipate a great deal of information changing frequently	

FIGURE 7.4 Searching and Screening Tool (Appendix C), Section III, part 2, answer key.

Part 5: Using the information you gathered above, spend some time developing a replicable search string for at least one database. Conduct the search and record the number of articles you found (see Figure 7.5).

What are the search strings and number of results from each database?		
Database	Search String	Number of Results
Medline (PubMed)	Search: (("Accidental Falls/prevention and control"[Mesh]) OR (FALL PREVENTION)) and (((ADULT) and (HOSPITAL*)) or (ADMITTED) and (Y_5[Filter])) **Filters:** in the last 5 years, Full text	1,896
CINAHL	MH "Accidental Falls/PC") AND adults AND hospital* Limiters – Full Text; Publication Date: 20190101-20241231	49

FIGURE 7.5 Searching and Screening Tool (Appendix C), Section III, part 3, answer key.

Learning Activity 7.3

Identify two ways the team can effectively screen the evidence from the searches.

Possible answers include:

- Establish inclusion and exclusion criteria for screening (i.e., date, population, language, intervention, outcome, or setting).
- Complete the task as a team with more than one reviewer looking at each article.
- Use screening software or a web-based program to track.
- Use a third reviewer to resolve conflicts over inclusion/exclusion.

Learning Activity 7.4

Complete the screening flow chart based on the following scenario:

The EBP team searched three databases—CINAHL, PubMed, and Embase—and found 230 articles to review. Team members additionally uncovered six articles through hand searching. The team reviewed the collected evidence and found and removed 23 duplicate articles. From a title and abstract screening of the remaining articles, five were removed because they were not in English, seven discussed children and not adults, 43 were not on topic, and 26 were excluded because they fell well outside the year limits. Subsequent full-text screening excluded 25 articles that used an alternative intervention that was not the focus of this project, 25 were based on children, and four were not retrievable as full text.

Answers:

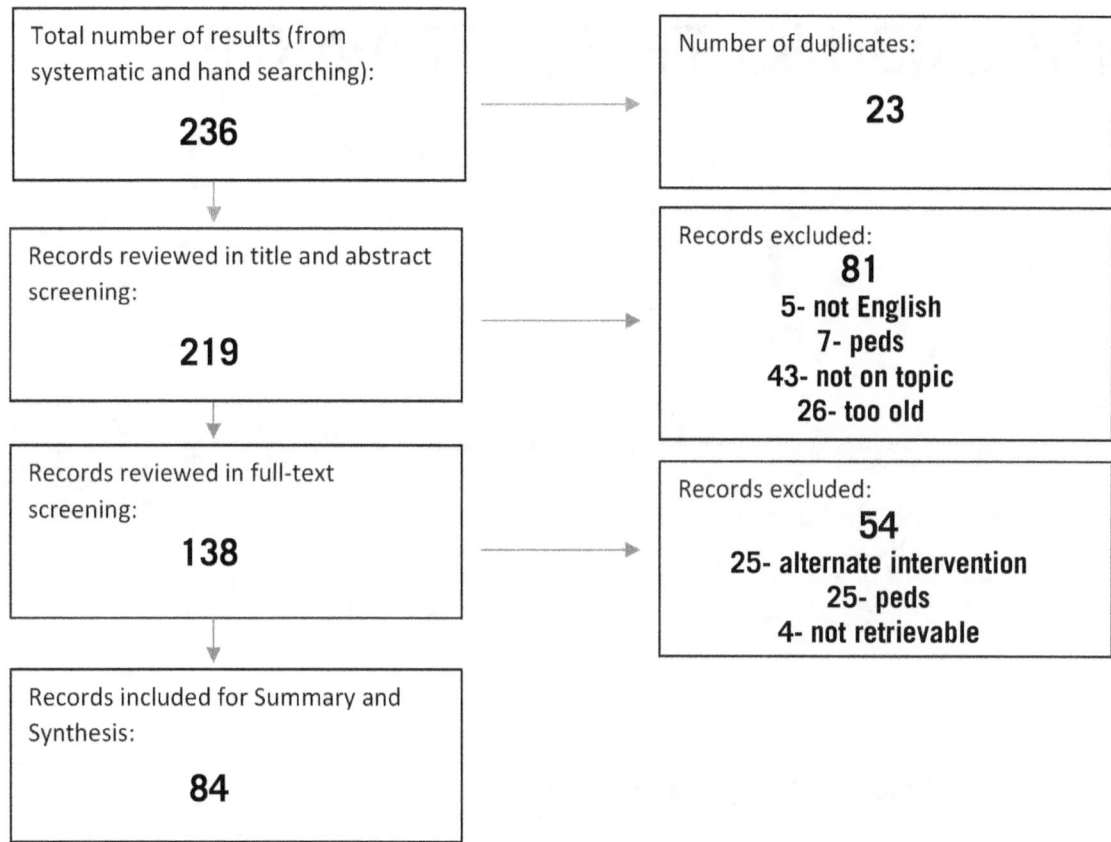

DISCUSSION QUESTIONS

1. What are the different types of literature searches, and how can an EBP team determine which type is most suitable for addressing their specific EBP question?

2. What strategies can EBP teams use to efficiently process and screen search results to ensure they are left with a manageable and accurate representation of the literature?

3. How does the selection between pre-appraised evidence and a comprehensive literature search affect the outcomes of an EBP project? What are the advantages and limitations of each approach?

4. In what ways might biases be introduced during the literature search and screening process, and what steps can the EBP team take to minimize these biases?

5. Why is it essential for EBP teams to be vigilant about potential biases in the evidence collection phase, and what impact could these biases have on the final recommendations and patient care outcomes?

8

EVIDENCE PHASE: APPRAISING THE EVIDENCE

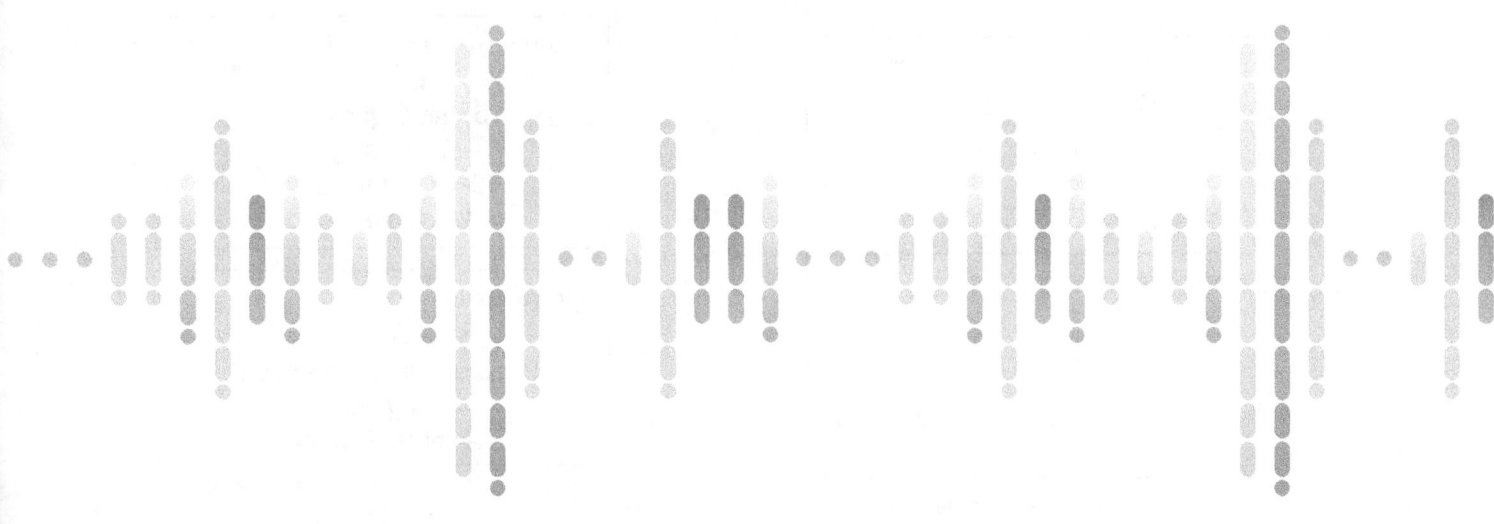

LEARNING OBJECTIVES

- 8.1 Describe the different paths EBP projects may take (understanding)

- 8.2 Differentiate between the different types of single-study evidence (analyzing)

- 8.3 Recognize evidence terminology and important considerations (understanding)

- 8.4 Appraise evidence using a guide (evaluating)

LEARNING ACTIVITIES

Before completion of the learning activities, learners are directed to do the following:

- Read Chapter 8

- Download the Appraisal Tool Selection Algorithm (Appendix D), Pre-Appraised Evidence Appraisal Tool (Appendix E1), Single Study Evidence Appraisal Tool (Appendix E2), Anecdotal Evidence Appraisal Tool (Appendix E3), and Evidence Terminology and Considerations Guide (Appendix F) (Hopkins.org/tools)

- Read Article 1: https://academic.oup.com/ageing/article/53/7/afae149/7716267

- Read Article 2: https://jamanetwork.com/journals/jamanetworkopen/fullarticle/2773051#google_vignette

- Read Article 3: https://www.the-hospitalist.org/hospitalist/article/36605/critical-care/how-can-hospitalists-help-reduce-harmful-in-hospital-patient-falls/

Learning Activity 8.1

Read the following summaries of five fictional articles. For each, use the Appraisal Tool Selection Algorithm (Appendix D) to determine 1) the level of support for decision-making and 2) which appraisal tool best suits the evidence at hand (see Figure 8.1).

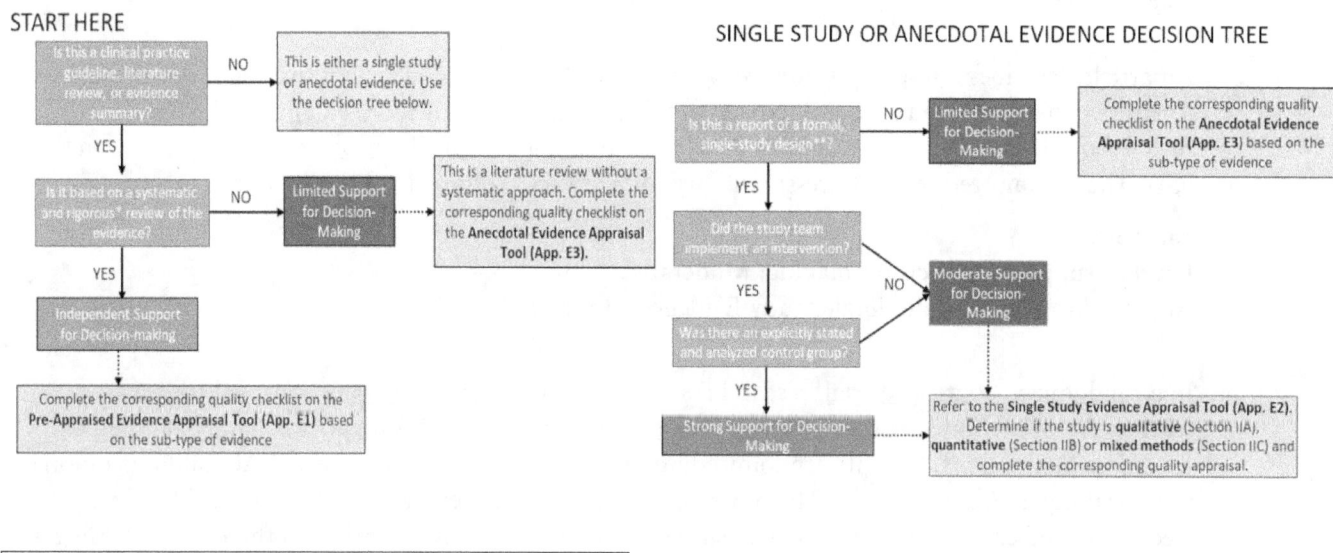

FIGURE 8.1 Appraisal Tool Selection Algorithm (Appendix D).

> **Facilitator Note:** The words and phrases underlined below are helpful hints for determining the type of evidence and using the selection algorithm.

1. A <u>systematic review</u> with meta-analysis explores the use of artificial intelligence (AI) in healthcare. The authors all appear to be experts in the field of study. Twenty-five articles were included in the review, and <u>definitive inclusion/exclusion criteria</u> were established. The <u>quality</u> of the studies included was <u>clearly established.</u> The researchers reported <u>following PRISMA guidelines</u> to conduct the review.

    Answers:
    Level of support for decision-making: **Independent**
    Appraisal tool to consult: Pre-appraised Evidence Appraisal Tool (**E1**)

2. A journal article provides a <u>review of several studies</u> on nurses' use of AI. The author explores what is known about the topic and <u>provides a summary</u> of the evidence. No <u>formal process</u> or <u>protocol</u> for the review was provided. Twelve references were included, though <u>no analysis of their strengths or weaknesses</u> is evident. The author concludes with recommendations for further study and implications for practice.

    Answers:
    Level of support for decision-making: **Limited**
    Appraisal tool to consult: Anecdotal Evidence Appraisal Tool (**E3**)

3. An article describes <u>a research study</u> using AI to determine the frequency of turning for ICU patients. The researchers reported a <u>"quasi-experimental study design"</u> that received <u>approval from the ethical review board.</u> The study team used an AI system to develop a <u>turning protocol</u> for <u>all patients</u> in the ICU. They monitored rates of pressure injury for six weeks following initiation of the protocol.

    Answers:
    Level of support for decision-making: **Moderate**
    Appraisal tool to consult: Single Study Evidence Appraisal Tool (**E2**)

4. In a <u>randomized controlled trial</u>, researchers report receiving <u>ethical review approval</u> for a 12-week study of the impact of <u>AI-generated patient teaching materials</u> on patients' understanding of <u>discharge instructions.</u> Patients randomized into the intervention group received AI handouts tailored to their unique medical history. The other patients received generic materials generated from the electronic medical record. Patients were surveyed at discharge, one month, and three months using a validated instrument.

    Answers:
    Level of support for decision-making: **Strong**
    Appraisal tool to consult: Single Study Evidence Appraisal Tool (**E2**)

5. An article provides details of an <u>organization's initiative</u> aimed at decreasing the time it takes for medications to be received on the unit once an order has been placed. AI software was used to read and verify the orders for accuracy, check the patient's record for any contraindications, and ensure the hospital supply of the medication/dosage. A pharmacist would then double-check the results and send the order to be filled. Both the pharmacist and the unit staff <u>reported improved efficiency.</u>

Answers:
Level of support for decision-making: **Limited**
Appraisal tool to consult: Anecdotal Evidence Appraisal Tool (E3)

Learning Activity 8.2

Differentiate the different types of single-study evidence. Complete the following table based on your readings.

FEATURE	RANDOMIZED CONTROLLED TRIAL	QUASI-EXPERIMENTAL	DESCRIPTIVE	QUALITATIVE
Type of Study	Experimental	**Experimental**	Observational	Exploratory
Randomization	**Yes**	**No**	No	No
Control Group	Yes	May or may not have	**No**	**No**
Purpose	Test cause-effect	**Evaluate effects without randomization**	Describe characteristics	**Explore experiences**
Data Type	**Quantitative**	**Quantitative, some qualitative**	**Quantitative and/or descriptive**	**Qualitative (text, narratives, themes)**
Strengths	**High internal validity, control over variables**	**Feasible in real-world settings when randomization is not possible**	**Good for baseline data, easy to conduct**	**Rich, deep understanding of human experience**
Limitations	**Expensive, ethical concerns, not always feasible**	**No full control over variables, weaker cause-effect inference**	**Cannot establish causality, limited by bias**	**Not generalizable, subject to researcher bias, time-consuming**

Learning Activity 8.3

Part 1: Define bias and differentiate it from quality assessment.

	DEFINITION	CONSIDERATIONS
Bias	Bias can be described as any systematic error introduced into a study (in design, conduct, or analysis) that leads to results that are not a true representation of the population or do not accurately reflect the original question.	Biases can cause the findings from studies or reviews to not accurately reflect the truth. There are many types of biases, and it is the responsibility of study teams and reviewers to make efforts to mitigate them and include these efforts in their report. Of note, the terms "quality assessment" and "bias assessment" are often used interchangeably but do not mean the same thing. Quality assessment looks at using safeguards to minimize bias.

Part 2: Using the definitions provided, identify the type of bias described.

1. Researchers developed a study to examine the effectiveness of a new drug. The sample only includes participants who volunteer to take part. These participants are more likely to be healthier and more motivated to follow the treatment protocol.

   Answer:
   Type of bias identified: **Selection**

2. Researchers are investigating a new product to promote sleep in hospitalized patients. A retrospective study on sleep products asks participants to recall the quality of their sleep in the past (within five years) and what sleep interventions were beneficial. Participants may not remember sleep disruptions or intervention used.

   Answer:
   Type of bias identified: **Recall**

3. A professor studies two teaching methods but the students in one group are taught by a more experienced teacher, while the other group is taught by a less experienced teacher.

   Answer:
   Type of bias identified: **Performance**

4. A sleep researcher only publishes studies where a treatment shows significant effects and not those studies where no effects were observed.

   Answer:
   Type of bias identified: **Publication**

5. In a qualitative study, the researcher conducts interviews with participants to explore their experiences with cancer treatment. While transcribing the commentary, the researcher overlooks any reports of negative interactions with physicians believing the patients' reports must be mistaken.

   Answer:
   Type of bias identified: **Observer**

Learning Activity 8.4

After reading the case study excerpt in Chapter 8 of the workbook, with your newly formed EBP team, you conduct a best-evidence search of the literature. Your team finds a pre-appraised article that answers the EBP question.

Part 1: After considering the information in the case study excerpt, read and appraise article 1 and complete the Pre-appraised Evidence Appraisal Tool (Appendix E1; see Figure 8.2).

Article 1: https://doi.org/10.1093/ageing/afae149

Pre-Appraised Evidence Appraisal

Fill in this data collection table after completing the suitability and quality assessments below.						
Article Number	Author, date, title	Type of pre-appraised evidence	Topic or intervention	Population	Setting	Recommendations that answer the EBP question
1	McKercher et al., 2024, Hospital falls clinical practice guidelines: a global analysis and systematic review	Systematic review without meta-analysis	Fall prevention	Adults	Hospital, in-patient	• Scored screening tools are no longer recommended; instead, a comprehensive fall risk assessment is recommended. • Individual interventions, such as patient education, staff training, use of assistive devices, exercise, environmental adaptations, and safe footwear are still consistently recommended. • Multifactorial interventions are recommended but must vary according to patient needs.

*For definitions of terms in **bold print** see **Appendix F: Evidence Terminology and Considerations Guide**

Section I: Suitability

Only complete this section if you are using this evidence as potential independent support for decision-making. **If you gathered this evidence in an exhaustive search, skip to Section II: Quality Appraisal.**

	Yes	No	Unclear	N/A
Is the topic or intervention the same or similar to the topic of interest?	X			
Is the population the same or similar to your population of interest?	X			
Is the setting the same or similar to your setting of interest?	X			
If applicable, are the **outcomes** the same or similar to your **outcomes** of interest?				X
How recent are the references (*provide date*)?	1997-2024			
Are the references recent enough to be reasonably applied to the practice setting (this will depend on the intervention and changing nature of the topic at hand)	X			
Notes: A total of 88 references were used, ranging in dates from 1997 – 2024 (31 years). However, 75% (66/88) were published within the past 10 years (2014 – 2024).				

*For independent support for decision-making, all responses must be YES. If the topic, population, setting, or outcome is similar, but not the same, include in the notes section the team's rationale for how the provided information can be reasonably compared to the elements in the team's EBP question. **If suitable, complete the corresponding quality assessment below.**

If the evidence is not fully suitable, but it informs the EBP question, complete the appraisal below. If the quality is adequate, this is strong support for decision-making, record the information on Appendix G: The Individual Evidence Summary Tool.

FIGURE 8.2 Pre-appraised Evidence Appraisal Tool (Appendix E1), answer key.

continues

Clinical Practice Guidelines	Yes	No	Unclear	N/A
1. Is the review group made up of experts who have proven expertise or skills related to the topic?				
2. Is the target population of the recommendations clear?				
3. Is the process for making the recommendations provided (e.g. evidence review, reaching consensus)?				
4. Are recommendations clear and complete (including a level of certainty/confidence)?				
	Yes	No	Unclear	N/A
5. Was there an external, peer-review of the guidelines?				
6. Does the level of certainty/confidence of each of the recommendations align with the evidence used to support them?				
7. Are funding and conflicts of interest addressed?				

If No → Exclude, set aside, and note exclusion for tracking

Complete the below checklist to determine the quality of the literature review used to generate the guidelines

Literature Reviews with a Systematic Approach (LRSAs)	Yes	No	Unclear	N/A	Notes
Background/Introduction					
1. Is a logical background and rationale for the review explained regarding current literature?	X				Found on Pg. 2 "Background" section
2. Is the review question clear?	X				Not a question but a statement, last paragraph of background section.
Methods					
1. Did the review follow a model or guideline (e.g. PRISMA, AMSTAR II, etc.)?	X				Found on Pg. 2 "Methods" section
2. Do the authors clearly state what they are trying to measure or describe?	X				Found on Pg. 2 "Background" section
3. Was the literature search thorough and could it be replicated (this includes providing keywords, inclusion/exclusion criteria, and at least 2 formal databases searched)?	X				Found on Pp. 2-3 "Search strategy" section
4. Was there an independent double-check system in the review process (this includes an independent assessment for eligibility, critical appraisal, and data extraction by at least two reviewers)?	X				
5. Was the quality of each included study formally assessed and listed?	X				Found on Pg. 3 "Quality appraisal", "Critical analysis", and "Confidence"
6. Was the risk of introducing bias into the literature selection and review minimized?	X				Understood by the use of multiple reviewers as mentioned several places on pg. 3
7. If applicable, were data pooling (meta-analysis or meta-synthesis) methods clear and appropriate?				X	
8. In addition to the items above, did the authors answer all of your questions about how they conducted their review [include notes about additional concerns]?	X				
Results					
1. Was there a flow diagram that included the number of studies eliminated at each stage of the review?	X				Found on Pg. 4
2. Were details of included studies provided (e.g. design, sample, methods, results, outcomes, limitations, the strength of evidence)?	X				
3. If applicable, are themes identified?	X				Evident in narrative beginning on pg. 3 and in
4. If applicable, are statistics shown clearly?				X	
	Yes	No	Unclear	N/A	
Discussion					
1. Does the discussion match what is reported in the results section?	X				
2. Do the authors examine what they found and compare it to other literature on the topic?	X				Beginning on Pg. 6
3. Are limitations included with an explanation of how they were handled?	X				
4. Do the authors provide implications of their study for practice and future investigation?	X				
General					
1. Is all the information in the paper congruent (consistent throughout the aims, methods, results, and discussion sections)?	X				
2. Are funding and conflict(s) of interest addressed?	X				Found on Pg. 9

Consider all of your responses above. Do you think the quality of this article is adequate to provide independent support for decision-making?

☒ Yes → Include, complete data collection table on page 1
☐ No → Exclude, set aside, and note exclusion for tracking

FIGURE 8.2 Pre-appraised Evidence Appraisal Tool (Appendix E1), answer key (cont.).

After reading the case study excerpt, suppose that—after a best-evidence search of the literature—your team did not find a pre-appraised article that answers the EBP question. Your team moves forward with an exhaustive literature search. Your team finds a total of 84 articles that answer the EBP question, including both single study and anecdotal evidence.

Part 2: After considering the information in the case study excerpt, use the Appraisal Tool Selection Algorithm (Appendix D; refer to Figure 8.1) to determine the level of support for decision-making and the appropriate appraisal tool to use to appraise Articles 2 and 3 and mark your answers on the following chart.

Article 2: https://jamanetwork.com/journals/jamanetworkopen/fullarticle/2773051#google_ vignette

Article 3: https://www.the-hospitalist.org/hospitalist/article/36605/critical-care/how-can-hospitalists-help-reduce-harmful-in-hospital-patient-falls/

ARTICLE #	ARTICLE OVERVIEW	LEVEL OF SUPPORT FOR DECISION-MAKING	EVIDENCE APPRAISAL TOOL
2	Article 2 discusses a study described as a nonrandomized controlled trial. A nurse-led fall prevention toolkit was implemented in 14 hospital units at three academic medical centers. Each unit served as its own control; researchers compared the rates of falls and falls with injury from a 21-month preintervention period to a 21-month postintervention period. Researchers report receiving a waiver of informed consent from the ethical review board owing to the quality-improvement nature of the intervention.	Strong	Single Study Evidence Appraisal Tool (Appendix E2)
3	Article 3 provides a review of two doctors' opinions about fall prevention strategies in adults in two different hospitals. The author provides a brief overview of what is known about the topic and then dives into each doctor's personal experience. No formal process or protocol was provided for any of the fall prevention strategies discussed by either doctor.	Limited	Anecdotal Evidence Appraisal Tool (Appendix E3)

Part 3: Appraise Articles 2 and 3 using the appropriate evidence appraisal tool. Fill out one appraisal tool for each article (see Figures 8.3 and 8.4).

Answer: Article 2:

Single Study Evidence Appraisal Tool

Section I: Level of Support for Practice Change

Complete the decision tree below to determine the level of support for practice change

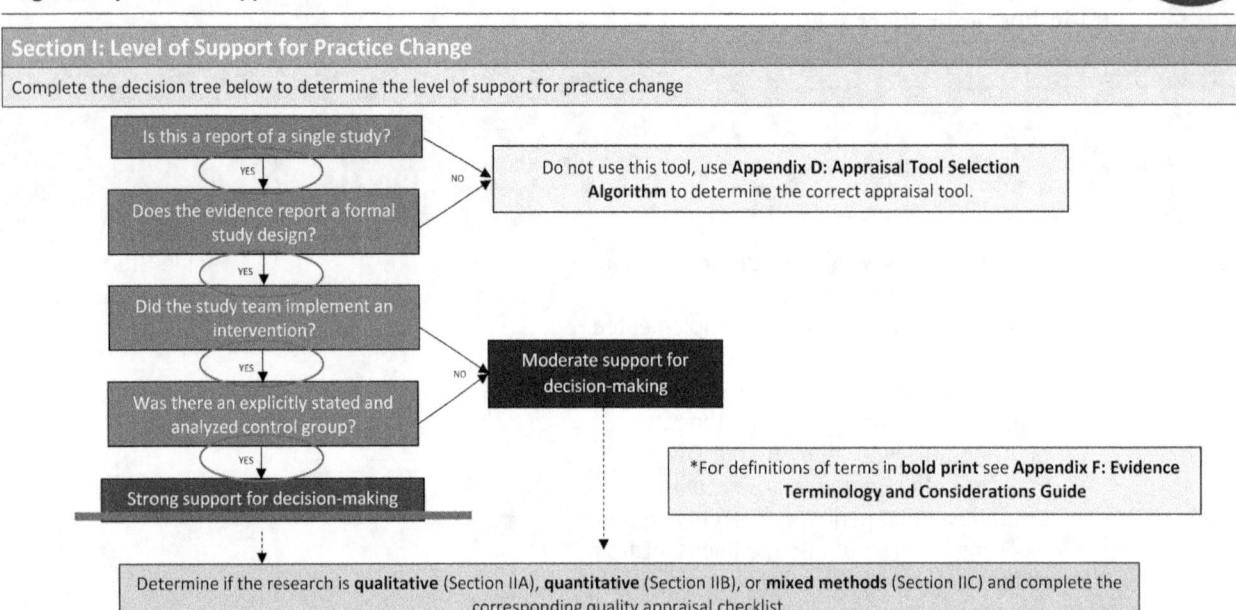

*For definitions of terms in **bold** print see **Appendix F: Evidence Terminology and Considerations Guide**

Determine if the research is **qualitative** (Section IIA), **quantitative** (Section IIB), or **mixed methods** (Section IIC) and complete the corresponding quality appraisal checklist.

Fill in this data collection table after completing the quality assessment below (see Instructions in **Appendix G2: Individual Evidence Summary Tool** for more information)

Article Number	Author, date, title	Type of evidence	Population, size, and setting	Intervention	Findings that help answer the EBP question	Measures used	Limitations	Level of support for decision-making
2	Dykes et al., 2020, Evaluation of a patient-centered fall-prevention tool kit to reduce falls and injuries: A randomized controlled trial	Single study, quantitative, quasi-experimental	37,231 adult patients over 277,644 patient-days 14 adult medical units at 3 academic medical centers Boston and NYC	Fall Tailoring Interventions for Patient Safety (TIPS) toolkit, which links nurse-identified risk factors from the Morse Fall Scale to appropriate preventative interventions. The TIPS tool kit is displayed at the bedside and reviewed with the patient and family at admission and during each shift. Both high-tech and low-tech modalities were used: laminated poster, integrated into the electronic health record (EHR), and an electronic bedside screen.	Engaging patients and families in the fall-prevention care plan has shown to significantly reduce rates of falls, particularly in adults younger than 65 Engaging patients and families in the fall-prevention care plan has shown to significantly reduce rates of falls with injury, particularly in adults 65 or older Both high-tech and low-tech tools can be used to facilitate patient engagement, allowing for easy integration into existing clinical workflows in diverse hospital settings	Primary: Rate of patient falls per 1000 patient days Secondary: Rate of patient falls with injury per 1000 patient days	Extensive refining of processes during the early phases of the project could have impacted outcomes. Allowing clinicians to select the tool modality, either high-tech or low-tech, limited the ability to randomize. 12/14 units were from site 1. Site 2 and 3 only involved a single unit. Older references were used.	Strong

	Yes	No	Unclear	N/A
2. Are **themes or patterns** identified clearly?				
3. Do the authors provide enough quotations, detailed observations, or other proof to support their findings?				
Discussion				
1. Does the discussion match what is reported in the results section?				
2. Do the authors examine what they found and compare it to other literature on the topic?				
3. Are **limitations** included with an explanation of how they were handled?				
4. Do the authors provide implications of their study for practice and future investigation?				
General				
1. Is all the information in the paper **congruent** (consistent throughout the aims, methods, results, and discussion sections)?				
2. Are funding and **conflicts of interest** addressed?				
Consider all of your responses above. Do you think the quality of this article is adequate to provide dependable information to answer your EBP question?	☐ Yes → *Include, complete data collection table on page 1* ☐ No → *Exclude, set aside, and note exclusion for tracking*			

Section IIB: Quantitative Evidence

	Yes	No	Unclear	N/A
Introduction/Background				
1. Is a logical background and rationale for the study explained using **current** literature?	X				*Introduction pp. 1-2*
2. Is the purpose/objective of the study clear? *P. 3 The goal of the trial…"*	X			
Methods				
1. Is the **study design** clearly stated? *Under Methods- pp 3-4 "Overall Design"*	X			
2. Is the **study setting** clearly described (including location, dates, and other important details) to enhance **generalizability**? *P. 4 Unit Selection and Participants*	X			
3. Is the process for recruiting participants (**sampling**) explained clearly and does it match with the study aim(s)? *Based on previous work other phases of the project*	X			
4. Do **eligibility** criteria (rules for who can join the study) make sense and are they easy to understand?	X			
5. Is the **sample size powered** adequately (a calculation or c many participants or observations to include)?	*The authors enrolled every patient from the participating units (mentioned in the abstract). Since they included the entire relevant population, a power analysis is not needed.*			
6. Did the authors clearly state what they wanted to measure? *P. 4 Outcomes- "The primary outcome measure…"*				

	Yes	No	Unclear	N/A
7. Are the **data collection** methods clear and appropriate (this includes how they gathered and recorded the information)?	X			
a) If applicable, were all the tools **reliable**?	X				*P. 4 Study Design and Intervention*
b) If applicable, were all the tools **valid**?	X			
8. Are the methods to analyze the data well explained (this includes what computer programs they used, how they made calculations, or anything else they did to explore the data)?	X			
9. If applicable, are the intervention(s) clearly described?	X			
10. If there was **randomization**,				
a) Was true **randomization** used to put people in the **control** and **intervention** groups?				X
b) Other than the intervention being studied, were the **intervention** and **control** groups treated similarly?				X
11. Is there information on the **ethical review** provided?	X				*P. 4 top of page "The study was approved…"*
12. In addition to the items above, did the authors answer all of your questions about how they conducted their study [include notes about additional concerns]?	X			
Results/Findings				
1. Do the findings make sense and are they easy to understand?	X			
2. Are characteristics of the participants provided (this may include demographics or other important details about the participants or things being studied)?	X				*Pp. 5-6 Results*
3. If applicable, was the survey **response rate** provided?				X
4. If applicable, are **attrition** rates provided (this includes how many people remained with the study at each stage)?				X
5. Is data provided for each item the authors stated they wanted to measure?	X			
6. If applicable, are the baseline characteristics of the **intervention** and **control** groups similar?	X				*Pp. 5-6 Results*
7. Are any statistics shown clearly?	X			
Discussion				
1. Does the discussion match what is reported in the results section?	X				*Discussion p. 7*
2. Do the authors examine what they found and compare it to other literature on the topic?	X			
3. Are **limitations** included with an explanation of how they were handled?	X				*Strengths and Limitations p. 7-8*
4. Do the authors provide implications of their study for practice and future investigation?	X			

	Yes	No	Unclear	N/A
General				
1. Is all the information in the paper **congruent** (consistent throughout the aims, methods, results, and discussion sections)?	X			
2. Are funding and **conflicts of interest** addressed?	X				*Pg. 9*
Consider all of your responses above. Do you think the quality of this article is adequate to provide dependable information to answer your EBP question?	☒ Yes → *Include, complete data collection table on page 1* ☐ No → *Exclude, set aside, and note exclusion for tracking*			

FIGURE 8.3 Single Study Evidence Appraisal Tool (Appendix E2), answer key for article 2.

Answer: Article 3:

Anecdotal Evidence Appraisal Tool

Fill in this data collection table after completing the quality assessment below (see Instructions in **Appendix G2: Individual Evidence Summary Tool** for more information).

Article Number	Author, date, title	Type of evidence	Population, size, and setting	Intervention	Findings that help answer the EBP question	Measures used	Limitations	Level of support for decision-making?
3	Beresford, 2024, How can hospitalists help reduce harmful in-hospital patient falls?	Anecdotal, expert opinion	2 physicians from 2 hospitals, one in Colorado and one Indiana	No intervention was implemented. The author provided a brief overview of what is known about fall prevention, and then discussed each physicians' personal experiences and opinions with fall prevention strategies.	It is believed that hospitalists can play a role in fall prevention by 1) creating a culture that is supportive of quality and safety 2) adjusting prescribing of high-risk medications and 3) engaging patients and families in the fall prevention care plan. Using a mobility technician, who is dedicated to mobilizing patients during their hospital stays, is a promising intervention	Fall rates	The article does not discuss limitations. Only consulting two people offers a very limited view of the topic. Only 9 references were used to describe the current state of the literature.	Limited

*For definitions of terms in **bold print** see **Appendix F: Evidence Terminology and Considerations Guide**

Section I: Quality Appraisal

Complete the checklist below for the corresponding sub-type of evidence. Note, the headers within each checklist are used for organization and may not match the exact language from the article or report being appraised

Expert Opinion, Position Statements, and Book Chapters	Yes	No	Unclear	N/A
Author(s) expertise				
1. Does the author(s) know about the topic of interest as evidenced by previous relevant professional or academic **affiliations**, related education/training their **expertise**? *(The author is a freelance medical journalist with experience writing about medical topics. He consults with experts in the field to make recommendations.)*			X	
Purpose/objectives				
1. Is the purpose/objective(s) clearly stated?	X	p. 12		
Reference to evidence				
1. Is there a thorough reference to **current** literature on the topic? *(Found in several places throughout, for example under "Techniques and approaches")*	X			
2. Do the author(s) provide meaningful **analysis** (through insights or commentary) of existing evidence on the topic? *(Commentary throughout)*	X			
Summary/conclusions				
1. Is it clear and logical how the authors reached their conclusion(s)?	X			
2. Are recommendations clear? *(Yes and evidence regarding efficacy is mentioned as well)*	X			
	Yes	No	Unclear	N/A
General				
1. Are funding and **conflicts of interest** addressed?		X		

Consider all of your responses above. Do you think the quality of this article is adequate to provide dependable information to answer your EBP question?

☒ Yes → Include, complete data collection table on page 1
☐ No → Exclude, set aside, and note exclusion for tracking

FIGURE 8.4 Anecdotal Evidence Appraisal Tool (Appendix E3), answer key for article 3.

DISCUSSION QUESTIONS

1. What is the purpose of the appraisal process in EBP, and how does it contribute to the overall quality of the team's decision-making?

2. How should an EBP team approach the appraisal of different types of evidence, and what special considerations are necessary for each type?

3. What criteria can be used to assess the relevance, validity, and reliability of evidence during the appraisal process, and why are these criteria important for ensuring high-quality recommendations?

4. How does a well-conducted appraisal process prepare an EBP team for the steps of summarizing, synthesizing, and generating best-evidence recommendations? What are the potential risks of advancing without thorough appraisal?

5. Reflect on a time when evidence was appraised incorrectly or insufficiently. What impact might this have on patient care, and how can EBP teams avoid similar pitfalls in their appraisal process?

9

EVIDENCE PHASE: SUMMARY, SYNTHESIS, AND BEST-EVIDENCE RECOMMENDATIONS

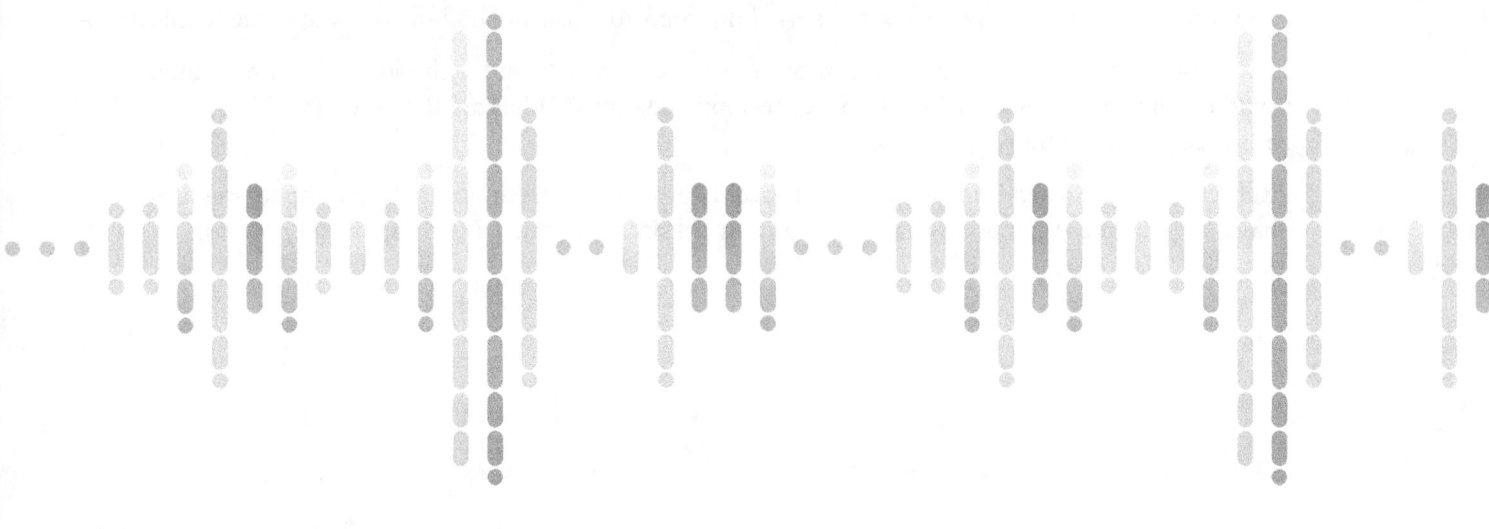

LEARNING OBJECTIVES

- 9.1 Differentiate between summary and synthesis (analyzing)
- 9.2 Develop a summary of the evidence (creating)
- 9.3 Develop a synthesis of the evidence (creating)
- 9.4 Select best-evidence recommendations (evaluating)

LEARNING ACTIVITIES

Before completion of the learning activities, learners are directed to do the following:

- Read Chapter 9
- Listen to the following podcast: https://podcasts.apple.com/us/podcast/ep-6-johns-hopkins-nursing-center-for-nursing-inquiry/id1478145611?i=1000448670865
- Download the Best-Evidence Summary Tool (Appendix G1), Individual Evidence Summary Tool (Appendix G2), and Summary, Synthesis, & Best-Evidence Recommendations Tool (Appendix H)

Learning Activity 9.1

Differentiate between summary and synthesis. Complete the following table.

	SUMMARY	SYNTHESIS
Definition	A restatement of key points	An integration of multiple sources forming a new understanding
Purpose	Provides an overview of existing information	To combine insights and develop new recommendations or conclusions
Content Focus	Highlights main ideas or findings	Integrates findings from various sources
Depth of Analysis	Generally superficial, presents information as is	More involved, includes a critical analysis and comparison of information
Use in EBP	To understand individual pieces of evidence	To understand the evidence as a whole and develop recommendations
Outcome	A snapshot of existing literature	New insights or actionable recommendations

Learning Activity 9.2

Using the evidence that you appraised in Learning Activity 8.4, summarize the evidence. Complete the Best-Evidence Summary Tool (Appendix G1; see Figure 9.1) and the Individual Evidence Summary Tool (Appendix G2; see Figure 9.2) as appropriate.

Section I: Pre-Appraised Evidence						
Complete the data collection tool below for all included pre-appraised evidence.						
Article Number	Author (organization), date, title	Type of pre-appraised evidence	Topic or Intervention	Population	Setting	Recommendations that answer the EBP question
1	McKercher et al., 2024, Hospital falls clinical practice guidelines: an analysis and systematic review	Systematic review without meta-analysis	Fall Prevention	Adults	Hospital, in-patient	• Scored screening tools are no longer recommended; instead, a comprehensive fall risk assessment is recommended. • Individual interventions, such as patient education, staff training, use of assistive devices, exercise, environmental adaptations, and safe footwear are still consistently recommended. • Multifactorial interventions are recommended but must vary according to the patient's needs.

FIGURE 9.1 Best-Evidence Summary Tool (Appendix G1), answer key.

Purpose: This tool collates information from the literature gathered during the exhaustive evidence search. It brings all of the data into a central document to help the EBP team with the next step of the EBP process, synthesis.

Complete the data collection tool below for all included evidence from the exhaustive evidence search										
Article number	Reviewer names	Author, date, and title	Type of evidence	Population, size, and setting	Intervention	Findings that help answer the EBP question	Measures used	Limitations	Level of support for decision-making	Notes to the team
2	AJ, KB	Dykes et al., 2020, Evaluation of a patient-centered fall-prevention tool kit to reduce falls and injuries: A randomized controlled trial	Quantitative, quasi-experimental	37,231 adult patients over 277,644 patient-days 14 adult medical units at 3 academic medical centers Boston and NYC	Fall Tailoring Interventions for Patient Safety (TIPS) toolkit, which links nurse-identified risk factors from the Morse Fall Scale to appropriate preventative interventions. The TIPS tool kit is displayed at the bedside and reviewed with the patient and family at admission and during each shift. Both	Engaging patients and families in the fall-prevention care plan has shown to significantly reduce rates of falls in adults younger than 65, and has shown to significantly reduce rates of falls with injury in adults 65 or older Both high-tech and low-tech tools can be used to facilitate patient engagement, allowing for easy integration into existing clinical	Primary: Rate of patient falls per 1000 patient days Secondary: Rate of patient falls with injury per 1000 patient days	Extensive refining of processes during the early phases of the project could have impacted outcomes. Allowing clinicians to select the tool modality, either high-tech or low-tech, limited the ability to randomize.	Strong	

#	Initials	Author, Year, Title	Design	Sample/Setting	Intervention	Findings	Measures	Limitations	Quality	
					high-tech and low-tech modalities were used: laminated poster, integrated into the electronic health record (EHR), and an electronic bedside screen. Each unit served as it's own control.	workflows in diverse hospital settings		12/14 units were from site 1. Site 2 and 3 only involved a single unit. Older references were used.		
3	AJ, KB	Beresford, 2024, How can hospitalists help reduce harmful in-hospital patient falls?	Anecdotal, expert opinion	2 adult hospitalists from 2 hospitals, one in Colorado and one Indiana	No intervention was implemented. The author provided a brief overview of what is known about fall prevention, and then discussed each physicians' personal experiences and opinions with fall prevention strategies.	It is believed that hospitalists can play a role in fall prevention by 1) creating a culture that is supportive of quality and safety 2) adjusting prescribing of high-risk medications and 3) engaging patients and families in the fall prevention care plan. Using a mobility technician, who is dedicated to mobilizing patients during their hospital stays, is a promising intervention	Fall rates	The article does not discuss limitations. Only consulting two people offers a very limited view of the topic. Only 9 references were used to describe the current state of the literature.	Limited	
4	MW, JA	Morris et al., 2024, Preventing hospital falls: Feasibility of care workforce redesign to optimize patient falls education	Quantitative, Randomized Control Trial	541 patients; 30 adult units in a hospital in Australia	The control group received usual care. The intervention group continued to receive usual care plus additional falls education delivered by an allied health assistant within 48 hours of admission. The allied health assistants received a 3-hour training, an education script, and practice in a simulated scenario.	It is feasible and safe for supervised assistants to educate hospital patients about how to prevent falling. Patient education, delivered by allied health assistants, was shown to reduce the overall number of falls, falls with injuries, and falls requiring an escalation of care; however, not significantly due to the limited number of falls. Spending greater time communicating and engaging with patients and families about safety and fall prevention can improve outcomes.	Primary: to assess feasibility and safety, as measured by (1) time from admission to education delivery (2) and cost. Secondary: to assess efficacy, as measured by (1) fall rate per 1000 patient days (2) falls with injury (3) falls requiring escalation of care	The study was not powered to detect a significant effect for fall rates. The intervention may not be suitable for hospitals that do not employ allied health assistants, limiting the external validity of the results. The education was only developed in English, limiting the ability to scale up the intervention throughout the healthcare system and other hospitals.	Strong	

FIGURE 9.2 Individual Evidence Summary Tool (Appendix G2), answer key.

continues

| | | icons, and alarms | | | and was shown to patients by trained volunteers on a tablet device. The video was available in 4 languages. The icons displayed individual patient risk factors and interventions. They were mounted above the head of the bed and updated every 12 hours by nurses. Each unit served as its own control. | The icons were not sustained because it was physically difficulty to access and update the flip chart above the patient's bed.

Authors suggest using whiteboards instead to increase adherence.

Patients and families were attentive and engaged with the video and trained volunteers.

A personalized approach for patient education should be used for each patient, depending on their risk factors

It is unknown if there is an ideal time to provide fall prevention education | Falls with serious injury per 1000 patient days | the same time as the study, which could have also contributed to the reduction falls

Since the volunteer administered the video, researchers were unable to determine if it was the conversation with the volunteer or the video that contributed to the reduction of falls

The authors did not report how many patients were enrolled in the study | | |

FIGURE 9.2 Individual Evidence Summary Tool (Appendix G2), answer key (cont.).

Learning Activity 9.3

Using the summary completed above, synthesize the evidence using the Summary, Synthesis, & Best-Evidence Recommendations Tool (Appendix H; see Figures 9.3 and 9.4). Be sure to note the degree of support for decision-making for those recommendations. Also provide the summary of evidence from Appendix G1.

Section I: Pre-Appraised Evidence						
Complete the data collection tool below for all included pre-appraised evidence.						
Article Number	Author (organization), date, title	Type of pre-appraised evidence	Topic or Intervention	Population	Setting	Recommendations that answer the EBP question
1	McKercher et al., 2024, Hospital falls clinical practice guidelines: an analysis and systematic review	Systematic review without meta-analysis	Fall Prevention	Adults	Hospital, in-patient	• Scored screening tools are no longer recommended; instead, a comprehensive fall risk assessment is recommended. • Individual interventions, such as patient education, staff training, use of assistive devices, exercise, environmental adaptations, and safe footwear are still consistently recommended. • Multifactorial interventions are recommended but must vary according to the patient's needs.

Purpose: This tool guides the EBP team through the process of synthesizing the pertinent findings from the Best Evidence or Individual Evidence Summary (Appendix G1 or G2) to create an overall picture of the body of the evidence related to the EBP question. The team analyzes the data in each category of support for decision-making, as well as any additional organizational approaches that bring further insights.

Section I: Findings from the Individual Evidence Summary	
Support for Decision-Making	**Synthesized Findings with Article Number(s)** *(This is not a simple restating of information from each individual evidence summary—see instructions)*
Strong Number of sources = 3	Engaging patients and families in the fall-prevention care plan can help gain buy-in for fall prevention measures and prevent patient falls (2, 4, 5). Methods to engage patients and families include visual displays of risk factors and preventative interventions (2, 5) and using a dedicated staff member to deliver a scripted fall prevention education (4, 5). Both high- and low-tech modalities can be used to engage with patients and families (2, 5). High-tech modalities include electronic displays, videos, tablet devices, integration with the electronic health record, etc. (2, 4, 5). Low-tech modalities include printed handouts, laminated posters, etc. (2, 5). To be successfully implemented, low-tech modalities must be easy to access in patient rooms and easily updated (2, 5). With appropriate training, a variety of disciplines can safely and feasibly engage patients and families, including nurses, unlicensed assistive personnel, and volunteers (2, 4, 5).
Moderate Number of sources = 0	
Limited Number of sources = 1	Engaging patients and families in the fall-prevention care plan can help gain buy-in for fall prevention measures and prevent patient falls (3). Interdisciplinary approaches, such as collaborating with pharmacists to review high-risk medications, or collaborating with physical therapy to mobilize patients during their hospital stay, can help prevent falls (3).

FIGURE 9.3 Summary, Synthesis, & Best-Evidence Recommendations Tool (Appendix H), Section I, answer key.

Learning Activity 9.4

From the synthesis, develop the best-evidence recommendations (see Figure 9.4), paying attention to the characteristics of the recommendations. Write the recommendations as recommendations statements such as:

- There is high certainty evidence supporting the use of warming blankets.
- There is reasonable-to-low certainty evidence to recommend that nurses take naps on the night shift.

Section II: Best-Evidence Recommendations	
The recommendations below are based on:	
☐ Pre-appraised evidence identified in a best evidence search → Record each recommendation in the corresponding evidence category in the table below based on the confidence/certainty listed in the clinical practice guidelines, evidence summary or literature review with a systematic approach	
☐ Evidence appraised by the EBP team from a targeted search to supplement the pre-appraised evidence (single studies with a formal study design) → Record any additional or altered recommendations to the pre-appraised evidence in the corresponding evidence category in table below. See instructions for more details.	
☒ Evidence appraised by the EBP team from an exhaustive search (single studies, anecdotal evidence and pre-appraised evidence that does not fully address the EBP question) → Record each recommendation in the table below based on the team's analysis and synthesis of information in Section I	
Characteristics of the Recommendation(s)	**Best-Evidence Recommendation(s)**
High certainty recommendations (Robust, well-documented, consistent & persuasive, based mostly on evidence that provides strong support for decision-making)	• The evidence recommends engaging patients and families in the fall-prevention care plan (2, 3, 4, 5). • Visual displaying risk factors and preventative interventions (2, 5) is a useful technique for engaging patients and families. • Using a dedicated staff member to deliver a scripted fall prevention education is another useful technique for engaging patients and families (4, 5). • The evidence endorses using both high-tech (e.g. electronic displays, videos, tablet devices, integration with the electronic health record, etc.) and low-tech modalities (printed handouts, laminated posters, etc.; 2, 4, 5) to engage patients and families. • If a low-tech modality is used, it is recommended that it be easy to access and update in the patient's room (2, 5). • The evidence indicates, with the proper training, multiple disciplines can safely and feasibly engage with patients and families in the fall prevention care plan, including nurses, unlicensed assistive personnel, volunteers, providers, and physical therapists (2, 3, 4, 5).
Reasonable certainty recommendations (Good, mostly compelling, consistent evidence, based mostly on evidence that provides moderate to strong support for decision-making)	
Characteristics of the Recommendation(s)	**Recommendation(s) Lacking Adequate Evidence**
Reasonable to low certainty recommendations (Good but conflicting evidence. Inconsistent results, based mostly on evidence that provides moderate support for decision making)	

FIGURE 9.4 Summary, Synthesis, & Best-Evidence Recommendations Tool (Appendix H), Section II, answer key.

DISCUSSION QUESTIONS

1. Why is a thorough understanding of evidence crucial to the success of an EBP project, and what risks might an organization face if changes are implemented based on incomplete or poorly understood evidence?

2. What are the key components of a robust synthesis of evidence, and how can these components ensure the development of high-quality, best-evidence recommendations?

3. How does critical thinking contribute to the evaluation and synthesis of evidence, and in what ways can this skill enhance the overall effectiveness of an EBP project?

4. In what ways should patient and provider preferences be considered when translating evidence into organizational practice? Why is it essential to integrate these preferences into the decision-making process?

5. Reflect on a scenario where organizational change was implemented based on weak evidence. What lessons can be learned from such experiences, and how can they inform future EBP projects to ensure more reliable and impactful outcomes?

10

TRANSLATION PHASE: TRANSLATION

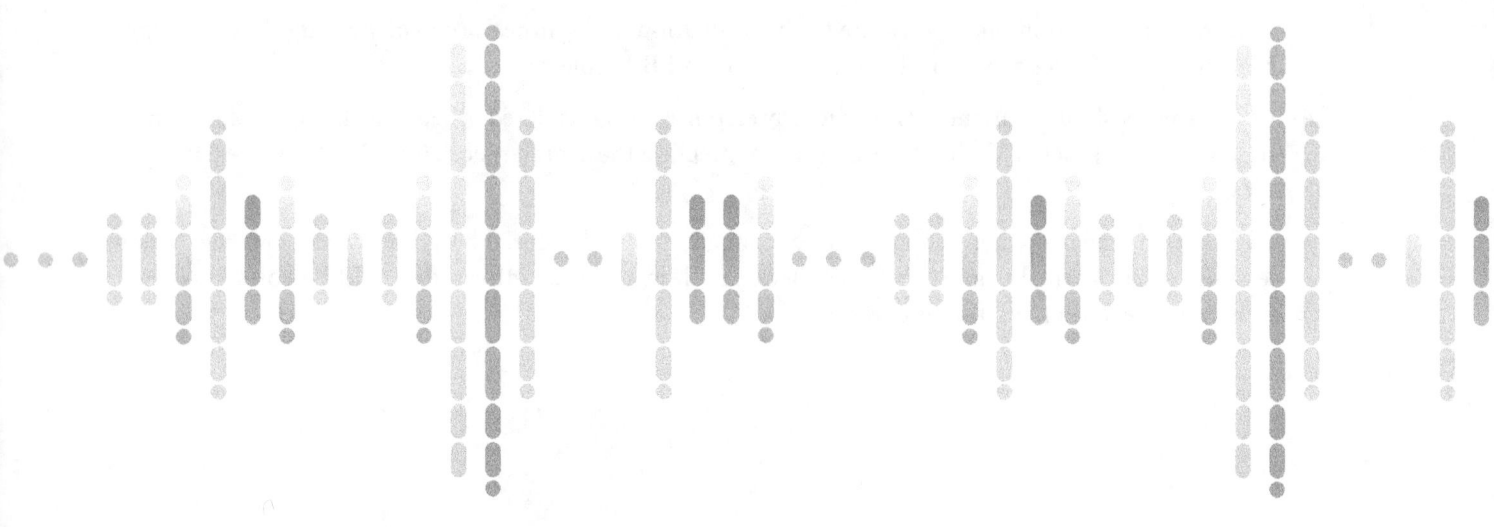

LEARNING OBJECTIVES

- 10.1 Differentiate between fit, feasibility, and acceptability (analyzing)
- 10.2 Develop organization-specific recommendations (creating)

LEARNING ACTIVITIES

Before completion of the learning activities, learners are directed to do the following:

- Read Chapter 10
- Download the Translation Tool (Appendix I)

Learning Activity 10.1

Differentiate between fit, feasibility, and acceptability. Complete the following table.

	FIT	**FEASIBILITY**	**ACCEPTABILITY**
Purpose	Ensures the recommendation is relevant and suitable for the target population or setting	Assesses the practicality of implementing the recommendations within existing constraints	Considers the perspectives and values of those affected by the recommendations
Key Questions	How well does the change align with existing practices? Values? Norms? Goals? Skills?	Is the change doable, and are barriers realistic to overcome? Is the practice environment ready for change? Are necessary materials or human resources available? Can the change be successfully implemented?	Do impacted groups find the change agreeable? Does leadership support the change and trust it is reasonable? Does the change align with organizational priorities?

Learning Activity 10.2

The case study excerpt in Chapter 10 of the workbook provides some insights about fit, feasibility, and acceptability around the best-evidence recommendations. Using this information, in a concise statement, develop an organization-specific recommendation that addresses the EBP question. Write your statement in the space below.

_____

_____

_____

BEST-EVIDENCE RECOMMENDATION	ORGANIZATION-SPECIFIC RECOMMENDATION
The evidence recommends engaging patients and families in the fall-prevention care plan (2, 3, 4, 5).	
Visually displaying risk factors and preventative interventions (2, 5) is a useful technique for engaging patients and families.	
Using a dedicated staff member to deliver a scripted fall prevention education is another useful technique for engaging patients and families (4, 5).	Your organization does not have the funding or current staff to hire a dedicated staff member to deliver fall prevention education. It is not recommended to move forward with this option.
The evidence endorses using both high-tech (e.g., electronic displays, videos, tablet devices, integration with the electronic health record, etc.) and low-tech (printed handouts, laminated posters, etc.) modalities to engage patients and families (2, 4, 5).	Your unit does not currently have and use the technology for a high-tech modality. Your organization also does not have the funding to purchase the technology needed to implement a high-tech modality. It is recommended that your unit uses a low-tech modality to engage patients.
If a low-tech modality is used, it is recommended that it be easy to access and update in the patient's room (2, 5).	It is recommended to hang fall prevention posters on the wall below each television. This location is easy to access by staff and to visualize by patients, family, and the care team.
The evidence indicates, with the proper training, multiple disciplines can safely and feasibly engage with patients and families in the fall prevention care plan, including nurses, unlicensed assistive personnel, volunteers, providers, and physical therapists (2, 3, 4, 5).	It is recommended to use a combination of nurses, unlicensed assistive personnel, and volunteers to engage patients and families with the fall prevention posters.

DISCUSSION QUESTIONS

1. What organizational considerations should be evaluated when deciding whether to implement a practice change based on evidence? How can factors like safety risk, fit, feasibility, and acceptability impact the success of the translation process?

2. Why is assessing organizational readiness critical before translating evidence into practice? What challenges might arise if this step is overlooked or insufficiently conducted?

3. What steps can an EBP team take to ensure that an intervention not only fits well within the organization but is also feasible and acceptable to stakeholders? Why are these considerations important for sustaining the practice change?

4. How can an EBP project benefit from using a structured framework to guide the translation process? What are some potential risks if a project moves forward without such a framework?

11

TRANSLATION PHASE: IMPLEMENTATION

LEARNING OBJECTIVES

- 11.1 Develop SMART goals to guide implementation (creating)
- 11.2 Identify appropriate metrics for a given project (understanding)
- 11.3 Complete a Work Breakdown Structure (WBS) outlining the implementation plan (understanding)

LEARNING ACTIVITIES

Before completion of the learning activities, learners are directed to do the following:

- Read Chapter 11
- Download the Implementation and Action Planning (A3) Tool (Appendix J) (Hopkins.org/tools)

Learning Activity 11.1

Using the recommendations in the case study excerpt from Chapter 11 of the workbook, identify two metrics appropriate for measuring the impact of the implementation.

Answers may vary but should match the recommendations, such as the following examples:

- Structure measure: the rate of fall prevention poster creation and installation
- Process measure: rate of completion of training on fall prevention signs, or rate sign usage
- Outcome measure: incident rate of falls measured as falls/1000 pt. days, falls with minor injury, and falls with major injury

Learning Activity 11.2

Using the case study excerpt from Chapter 8 of the workbook, write three SMART goals related to implementing the identified organization-specific recommendations.

Answers may vary but should match the outcome measures, such as the following examples:

- Structure measure: install fall prevention posters in 100% of bedsides in one month
- Process measure: achieve 90% staff compliance with sign usage in three months
- Outcome measure: reduce falls/1000 pt. days by 25% in six months

Learning Activity 11.3

Continuing with the case study excerpt, identify three high-level deliverables important to implementing the recommendations and ensuring success. Add them to the first column in the following table.

HIGH-LEVEL DELIVERABLE	ASSOCIATED TASKS AND SUB-TASKS	START DATE	END DATE	RESPONSIBLE PARTY	RESOURCES NEEDED
Create signs					
Train staff					
Inform patients and families					
Install signs					
Use signs					

DISCUSSION QUESTIONS

1. How does the TRIP model facilitate the translation of evidence-based recommendations into practice, and what are the key components of this implementation framework?

2. What role do goal-setting and timeline creation play in the success of an EBP project's implementation phase, and how can these elements be adapted when using other implementation frameworks?

3. What strategies can an EBP team employ to identify and mitigate barriers to implementation, and why is it important to address these challenges early in the process?

4. Why is a sustainability plan essential for EBP projects, and what factors should be considered to ensure that practice changes are maintained beyond project completion?

5. How can the use of communication strategies both within the EBP team and across the organization enhance the effectiveness of the implementation and contribute to long-term sustainability of the practice change?

12

ONGOING CONSIDERATIONS: COMMUNICATION AND DISSEMINATION

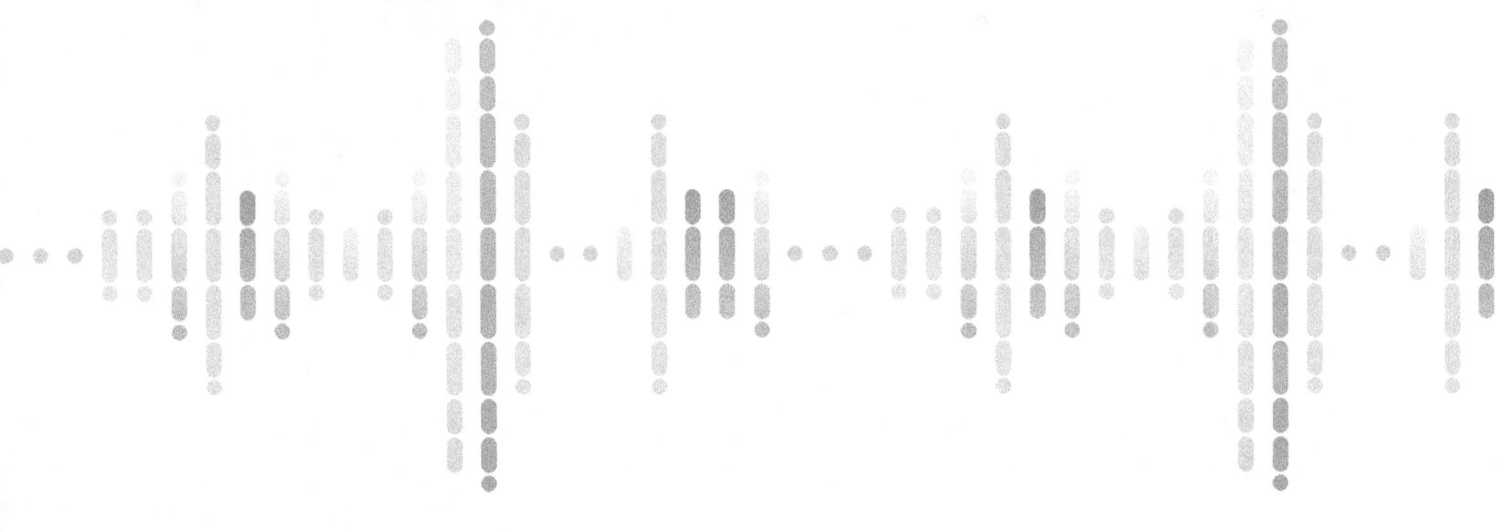

LEARNING OBJECTIVES

- 12.1 Identify the key components of a dissemination plan (understanding)
- 12.2 Consider the impacted groups identified previously, and craft messages according to the audience (Impacted Groups Analysis and Communication Resource) (creating)
- 12.3 Identify important components of an executive summary (understanding)

LEARNING ACTIVITIES

Before completion of the learning activities, learners are directed to do the following:

- Read Chapter 12
- Listen to the following podcast: https://podcasts.apple.com/us/podcast/ep-37-i-was-published-in-a-scholarly-journal-you/id1478145611?i=1000575529262
- Review the Impacted Groups Analysis and Communication Resource (Hopkins.org/resources)
- Download the JHEBP Publication Guide (Hopkins.org/resources)

Learning Activity 12.1

Identify the key components of a dissemination plan by filling in the following blanks.

Answer:

1. **Purpose:** will drive all other factors; examples may be to raise awareness, educate, share results
2. **Message:** should be clear, targeted, repeated several times, a call to action
3. **Audience:** messaging should be adjusted according to the recipients, their needs, and their background
4. **Timing:** consider when messages should be conveyed; requires repeated messaging
5. **Method:** approach to messaging should match the audience; a variety of channels should be used

Learning Activity 12.2

Considering the recommendations and plan, craft key messages and align with methods for the frontline nurses. Fill them out on the Impacted Groups Analysis and Communication Resource (see Figure 12.1) that follows.

Communication Planning			
Refer to this section to guide your communications to impacted individuals/groups throughout and after completing the EBP project.			
What is the purpose of the dissemination of the EBP project findings? (check all that apply) ☐ Raise awareness ☐ Change practice ☐ Inform impacted person(s) ☐ Promote action ☐ Engage impacted person(s) ☐ Other:_____ ☐ Change policy			
What are the 3 most important messages?			
We are pursuing a low-tech modality (fall prevention posters) to help prevent falls. Posters will be hung in all patient rooms below the TV. It is everyone's responsibility to engage patients and families about falls.			
Align key message(s) and methods with the audience:			
Audience	Key Messages	Method	Timing
Interdisciplinary impacted individuals/groups			
Organizational leadership			
Frontline nurses	Posters are an effective fall prevention tool when used with other interventions. We will be installing posters in all rooms and providing brief education. Nurses and techs are beneficial in providing education around fall prevention and the posters. We want to keep our patients safe.	Staff meeting, email, huddles	Weekly starting 2 weeks before start and continuing for three weeks into implementation; then as needed
Departmental leadership			
External community			
Other			

FIGURE 12.1 Impacted Groups Analysis and Communication Resource, answer key.

Learning Activity 12.3

Using the word bank provided, develop a logical outline for an executive summary.

ANSWER	WORD BANK
Current state of the problem	Project outcomes
Why change is needed	Sustainability plan
Overview of the project (align with strategic priorities)	Steps of the WBS
Implementation process	Organizational implications
Evaluation metrics	Evidence appraisal

Project outcomes	Why change is needed
Sustainability plan	Literature review
Organizational implications	Current state of the problem
	Overview of the project (align with strategic priorities)
	Evaluation metrics
	List of evidence reviewed
	PRISMA diagram
	Implementation process
	Schedule of outcome measurement

DISCUSSION QUESTIONS

1. What are the various forms of dissemination available for EBP projects, and how can the choice of dissemination method impact the reach and influence of the project's findings?

2. Why is dissemination considered an ethical responsibility for healthcare providers, and how is this reflected in professional codes of ethics such as those from the American Nurses Association and American Medical Association?

3. How can effective dissemination of EBP projects contribute to advancing the healthcare profession and improving patient care? What role does accessibility to knowledge play in this process?

4. In what ways does the unique perspective of clinically practicing healthcare providers enhance the value of disseminated EBP findings, particularly when it comes to realistic recommendations and best practices?

5. How can EBP teams use dissemination as a tool to advocate for specific patient populations or healthcare improvements? What considerations should be made to ensure that the advocacy efforts are both impactful and evidence-based?

PART 5
SAMPLE DNP SCHOLARLY PROJECT CURRICULUM OUTLINE

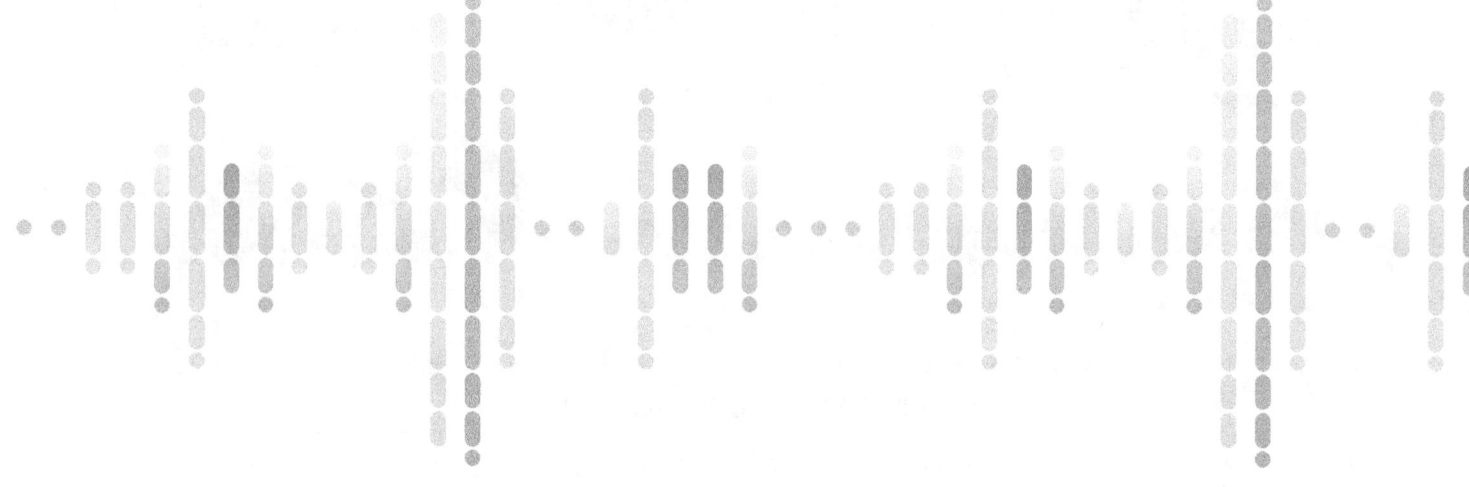

Aligned with the American Association of Colleges of Nursing (AACN) *Essentials* (2021), this content is structured to ensure the integration of core competencies in professional nursing education. The Johns Hopkins Evidence-Based Practice (JHEBP) Model for Nurses and Healthcare Professionals (Bissett et al., 2025; see Figure 5.1) provides the foundational framework for guiding evidence-based decision-making. Additionally, the curriculum draws on Melnyk and Fineout-Overholt's (2019) framework for implementing EBP competencies in academic settings, reinforcing a structured approach to EBP integration in graduate nursing programs. This alignment ensures that students develop proficiency in the Practice Question–Evidence–Translation (PET) process, bridging the gap between research and clinical practice while fostering a scholarly approach to improving patient outcomes.

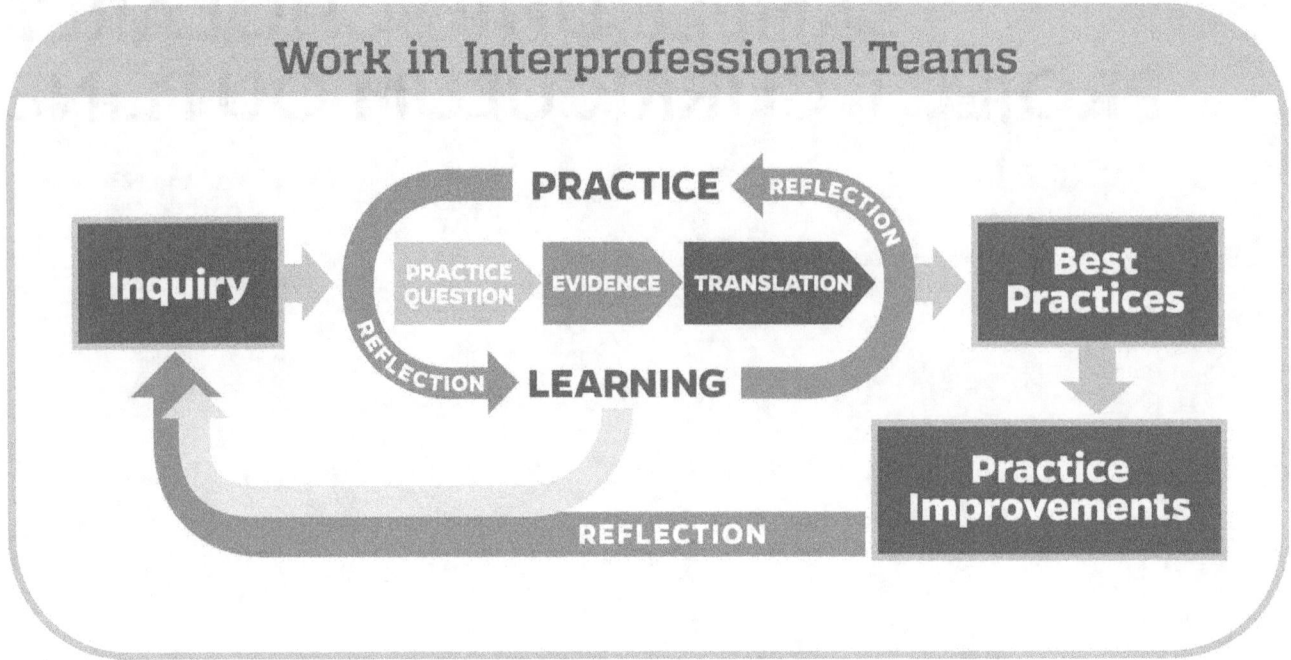

FIGURE 5.1 The JHEBP model (2025).

What follows is a structured curriculum outline for DNP scholarly projects—a sample plan of study for four to five courses, including 218 practicum hours.

PROJECT COURSE #1: PRACTICE QUESTION/PROBLEM STATEMENT AND IMPACTED GROUPS IDENTIFICATION

RN Competencies and Prerequisites: Learners Build Upon Baseline Knowledge and Professional Practice Application

- AACN *Essentials* entry-level (Level 1) Professional Nursing Education sub-competencies (AACN, 2021)
- EBP competencies #1–13 derived from pre-licensure RN program (Melnyk & Fineout-Overholt, 2019, p. 319)

Course Objectives

- Develop a clearly defined practice question and problem statement using the JHEBP model to guide clinical inquiry, ensuring alignment with the AACN *Essentials* (2021) competencies for EBP, quality improvement, and patient-centered care.
- Identify and engage key impacted groups in the DNP project by integrating strategic leadership principles from the AACN *Essentials* and applying analysis tools from the JHEBP model to facilitate collaboration, resource allocation, and sustainable practice change.
- AACN *Essentials* Level 2 Professional Nursing Education sub-competencies and domains (AACN, 2021, pp. 17–58)
- Melnyk & Fineout-Overholt, 2019, EBP Competencies in Graduate Programs #14–16

Course Activities/Assignments

- Review the organization's mission, vision and values and the Performance Improvement plan to understand the areas of focus.
- Identify a practice problem that aligns with the organizations focus to ensure alignment.
- Develop a practice question using the Question Development Tool (Appendix B).
- Practicum hours: 0–25 hours
- PET process: Learners identify project topic/focus/problem at a specific project site and for a specific population.
- Learners complete these worksheets to aid in focusing and narrowing their project approach:
  - EBP Project Steps and Overview (Appendix A)
  - Fishbone (see Figure 5.2 for an example; also oriented with concept map)
  - Question Development Tool (Appendix B)
  - Learners to identify their project team members/impacted groups (see the Impacted Groups Analysis and Communication Resource, available online at Hopkins.org/resources)
  - Hospital/unit impacted groups, community partners, primary care practices providers, health departments/clinics, legislative policy, nongovernmental organizations/nonprofit organizations, etc.

- Formulate problem statement/purpose of the project focus and choice:
  - Considerations: Does this look to be human subjects research (HSR), quality improvement (QI), and/or a process improvement (PI)?
  - Exploratory PET process: Will this be an individual or a team/group project?

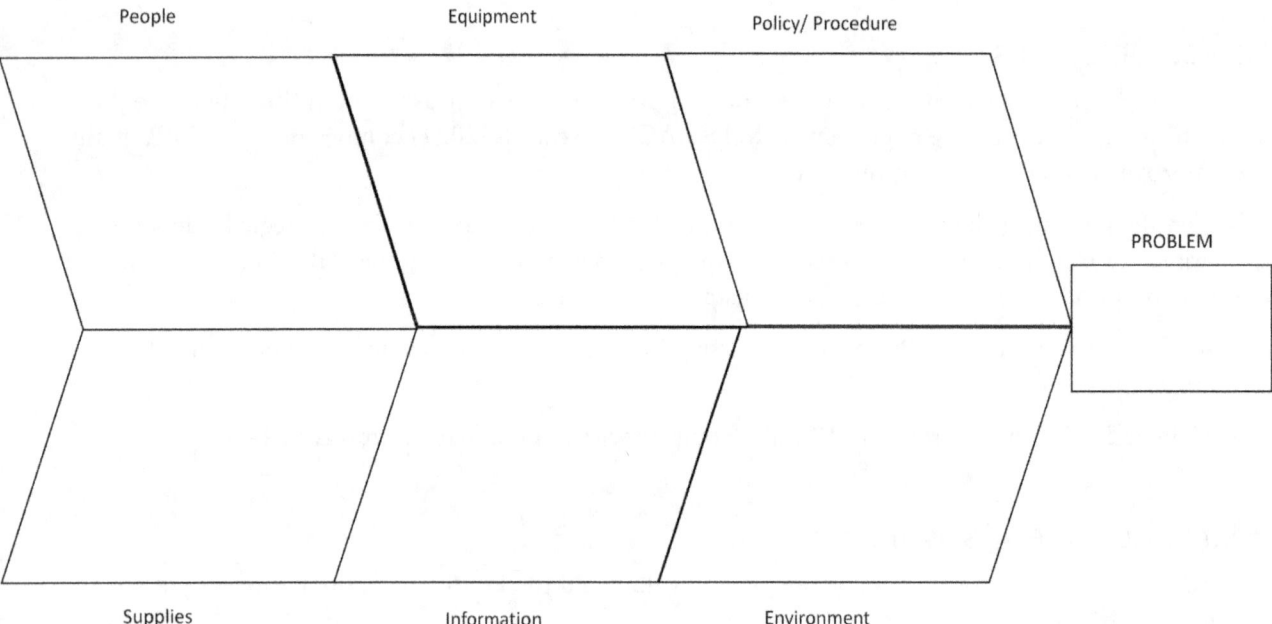

FIGURE 5.2 Fishbone template.

SAMPLE DNP PROJECT COURSE #1 SYLLABUS

Course Description

This is the first of five DNP project courses designed to provide students with a thorough understanding of the JHEBP module and how to implement from problem identification to data analysis. The first course will equip the student with the tools to identify, analyze, and address significant clinical practice problems. The students will learn evidence-based approaches and how to craft a high-impact clinical problem statement. The problems will be based on local data from the organization and supported by national and global data gleaned from going to the literature to substantiate the identified problem. The student will also learn about change and change readiness in an organization and how to complete an organizational assessment for readiness to change.

Students will explore how healthcare organizations identify and prioritize problems aligned with their mission, vision, values, and performance improvement plans. Students will be paired with an organizational team member to complete an organizational assessment, helping them identify relevant practice issues. This course emphasizes developing a spirit of inquiry and formulating well-crafted practice questions based on unanswered clinical questions, public health issues, or performance data. As the first step of the JHEBP PET process, students will work on the practice question phase, grounding their project in a problem that is well-suited for EBP intervention. Students will be exposed to local, national, and global data sources and gain an understanding of how to use data to identify practice problems. Students will explore the literature search to find evidence-based answers to their questions.

Course Learning Objectives (CLOs)

1. Craft a high-impact problem statement of importance to practice.
2. Use local, national, and global data to determine the significance of the problem.
3. Utilize a methodological approach for critical examination of the problem.
4. Synthesize biophysical, psychosocial, organizational, and public health literature to define a clinical issue of concern.
5. Apply disciplined habits of inquiry, reflection, and communication to the exposition of the practice problem.
6. Integrate principles of advanced nursing practice scholarship to improve equitable outcomes through organizational/system leadership, community/population health partnerships, policy/program evaluation, quality improvement processes, and translation of evidence into practice.
7. Integrate AACN *Essentials*.

12-WEEK SYLLABUS WITH SIX TWO-WEEK MODULES

Module 1 (Weeks 1–2): Identifying and Defining a Practice Problem

Learning Objectives
- Craft a high-impact problem statement of importance to practice (CLO1).
- Establish the relevance and scope of the problem.
- AACN *Essential* II (Organizational and Systems Leadership): Students identify organizationally relevant problems that align with mission and goals.
- AACN *Essential* IV (Scholarship for the DNP): Students develop a scholarly problem statement based on EBP needs.

Topics
- Principles of problem identification in healthcare
- The importance of practice-based problem-solving in nursing
- Crafting a compelling EBP problem statement

Activities
- Discussion on examples of clinical practice problems
- Workshop: Developing a problem statement

Assignment
Submit appropriate sections of Appendix B (Question Development Tool) by the end of week 2, including paper with sections on introduction and problem significance.

Module 2 (Weeks 3–4): Data-Driven Analysis of the Problem

Learning Objectives
- Use local, national, and global data to determine the significance of the problem (CLO2).
- AACN *Essential* IV (Scholarship for the DNP): Students critically assess data from multiple levels.
- AACN *Essential* VIII (Clinical Scholarship): Students use data-driven insights to understand and prioritize healthcare problems.

Topics
- Types of healthcare data: local, national, and global
- Using data to inform problem significance
- Ethical considerations in using health data

Activities

- Dataset Analysis: Analyze local, national, and global datasets to assess the scope of a clinical issue. Examples of local data include institutional performance metrics (e.g., infection rates, patient outcomes). National and global datasets may include sources like WHO and NIH.
- Local Data Discussion: Engage with your organization's Quality Department to discuss local data sources such as:
  - Joint Commission Core Measures
  - NDNQI for nursing-sensitive outcomes
  - Patient and Employee Experience data
  - Quality Indicators (e.g., readmission rates, hospital-acquired infections)
- Consider national metrics from AHRQ, CMS, and CDC for comparison.
- Literature Search: Conduct a literature search to gather national and global data related to your local problem.
- Guideline-Setting Organizations: Identify relevant guidelines from organizations like the ANA, AHA, and IDSA.
- Group Discussion: Collaboratively analyze the healthcare statistics and identify gaps between local and national/global benchmarks.

Assignment

Submit appropriate sections of Appendix B, integrating local, national, and global data along with clinical guidelines.

    Continue to develop paper and add background and section on local, national, and global data.

Module 3 (Weeks 5–6): Methodological Approaches to Problem Analysis

Learning Objectives

- Utilize a methodological approach for critical examination of the problem (CLO3).
- AACN *Essential* IV (Scholarship for the DNP): Students apply rigorous methods for problem analysis.
- AACN *Essential* VIII (Clinical Scholarship): Students utilize analytical methods for evidence-based problem examination.

Topics

- Research methodologies in nursing practice
- Quantitative vs. qualitative approaches
- Ethical issues in research

Activities
- Case Study: Apply both quantitative and qualitative methodologies to analyze nursing issues.
- Group discussion on the strengths and limitations of different methodologies.

Assignment

Continue to develop your paper and submit the proposed methodological approach for analyzing your identified problem.

Module 4 (Weeks 7–8): Literature Synthesis and Problem Contextualization

Learning Objectives
- Synthesize biophysical, psychosocial, organizational, and public health literature to define a clinical issue of concern (CLO4).
- AACN *Essential* VIII (Clinical Scholarship and Analytical Methods): Students integrate interdisciplinary literature to inform the clinical issue from an interdisciplinary perspective.
- AACN *Essential* IX (Mastery of Advanced Nursing Practice): Students expand and exhibit expertise by drawing on varied sources to inform problem definition.

Topics
- Conducting a comprehensive literature review
- Synthesizing evidence from biophysical, psychosocial, and organizational/public health fields
- Identifying gaps in research and practice

Activities
- Literature Review Exercise: Identify key sources for your problem.
- Group Discussion on synthesizing diverse literature.

Assignment

Continue to develop your paper and submit a four-to-five-page Literature Review, synthesizing biophysical, psychosocial, and public health factors related to your problem.

Module 5 (Weeks 9–10): Inquiry, Reflection, and Communication in Nursing Practice

Learning Objectives
- Apply disciplined habits of inquiry, reflection, and communication to the exposition of the practice problem (CLO5).

- AACN *Essential* VI (Interprofessional Collaboration): Students engage with mentors and team members to refine their inquiries.
- AACN *Essential* IX (Mastery of Advanced Nursing Practice): Students practice reflective and communicative skills crucial to advanced nursing practice.

Topics
- Reflective practice in advanced nursing
- Effective communication of complex clinical issues
- Inquiry-based learning in nursing practice

Activities
- Reflective Journaling: Reflect on the personal and professional relevance of your identified problem.
- Peer Feedback Sessions: Present your problem analysis and refine it through inquiry-based discussion.

Assignment
Submit a two-page Reflective Journal entry on the evolution of your problem statement and analysis based on inquiry and feedback.

Module 6 (Weeks 11–12): Advanced Nursing Practice Solutions for Equitable Outcomes

Learning Objectives
- Integrate principles of advanced nursing practice scholarship to improve equitable outcomes through leadership, community partnerships, policy/program evaluation, quality improvement, and evidence translation (CLO6).
- AACN *Essential* II (Organizational and Systems Leadership): Students address organizational needs through evidence based strategies.
- AACN *Essential* V (Quality and Safety): Students incorporate quality and safety principles in evidence translation.
- AACN *Essential* VIII (Clinical Scholarship and Analytical Methods): Students translate research into actionable plans.
- AACN *Essential* IX (Mastery of Advanced Nursing Practice): Students contribute to improved health outcomes through EBP leadership.

Topics
- Leadership and partnership for implementing solutions
- Policy and program evaluation
- Translating evidence into practice for quality improvement

Activities
- Case Studies: Review examples of successful quality improvement initiatives.
- Simulation: Conduct a policy/program evaluation exercise in a healthcare setting.

Assignment

Submit final paper including all sections from Modules 1–5: introduction, background, significance, local, national, and global data, potential solutions to problem, literature review, detailed problem statement, and completed Appendix B.

Resources

Agency for Healthcare Research and Quality (AHRQ): Resource for clinical guidelines, healthcare quality measures, and data to inform quality improvement projects (https://www.ahrq.gov/)

Centers for Medicare & Medicaid Services (CMS): Offers data and resources related to healthcare performance standards and quality improvement (https://www.cms.gov/)

National Database of Nursing Quality Indicators (NDNQI): A comprehensive resource for nursing-sensitive outcome measures (https://www.pressganey.com/platform/ndnqi/)

World Health Organization (WHO): A global resource for health data, policy guidelines, and evidence-based recommendations (https://www.who.int/)

Evaluation and Grading

- Question Development Tool, Problem Introduction (Module 1): 10%
- Question Development Tool, Data Analysis Report (Module 2): 15%
- Methodological Approach Paper (Module 3): 15%
- Literature Review Paper (Module 4): 20%
- Reflective Journal Entry (Module 5): 10%
- Final Paper and Appendix B (Module 6): 30%

PROJECT COURSE #2: EXPLORING THE EVIDENCE

Practice Question → **Evidence** → **Translation**

RN Competencies and Prerequisites: Learners Build Upon Baseline Knowledge and Professional Practice Application

Course Objectives

- Critically evaluate and synthesize existing literature using the JHEBP literature review tools and the PRISMA framework, applying data-driven methodologies to identify evidence-based solutions for their clinical inquiry.
- Explore and analyze local, national, and global databases to compare data and set benchmarks for project.
- Refine project AIMS using the SMART format and assess organizational readiness for EBP implementation by collaborating with their organizational mentor, ensuring alignment with clinical priorities and feasibility for practice change.
- Learners can now formulate Appendix H in the textbook.
- Continuation of achieving Melnyk & Fineout-Overholt EBP Competencies in Graduate Programs: #14–16.

Course Activities/Assignments

- Practicum hours: 0–25 hours
- Learners explore various EBP translational models (KTA, Iowa, etc.) or use the organization's translational EBP model for the project.
- Learners query and engage with the project site and impacted groups for microdata evidence supporting the need for an EBP project to improve patient care outcomes at that site and for the specified population. Learners compare this to the known micro and macro evidence.
- Learners identify clinical experts/leaders specific to the project topic.
- Learners explore the literature for evidence of current and up-to-date best practices and EBP methodologies, recommendations, and/or guidelines related to the project problem or topic focus.

- Learners complete these worksheet tools from the textbook:
    - Pre-Appraised Evidence Appraisal Tool (Appendix E1)
    - Single Study Evidence Appraisal Tool (Appendix E2)
    - Anecdotal Evidence Appraisal Tool (Appendix E3) for systematic searches (group work)
- Collaborating course: Integrative Review course (see Appendix G2, Individual Evidence Summary Tool, in the textbook)

SAMPLE DNP PROJECT COURSE #2 SYLLABUS

Connecting the Evidence for Project Translation and Organizational Readiness for Change

Course Description

Building on their initial practice question, students will dive into the evidence review process, using data-driven methodologies to uncover evidence-based solutions. This course guides students in performing a thorough literature review with the JHEBP literature review tool and PRISMA framework, allowing them to evaluate the body of evidence. Students will refine project AIMS using the SMART format and assess the organization's readiness for implementing evidence-based changes, staying in close contact with their organizational mentor. The course will emphasize integrating evidence to create a beginning project plan, laying the groundwork for a successful EBP initiative within the clinical setting.

Key JHEBP Tools: Appendix G, Appendix H, Appendix I, Appendix A

Competency-Based Assessment: Integrative review paper with project AIMS and a preliminary project plan

Course Learning Objectives (CLOs)

1. Conduct a comprehensive literature review utilizing the JHEBP literature review tool and PRISMA framework.
2. Evaluate the body of evidence to determine evidence-based solutions for identified clinical issues.
3. Refine project AIMS using the SMART format, aligning with organizational goals.
4. Assess organizational readiness for implementing evidence-based changes, working closely with an organizational mentor.
5. Develop a preliminary project plan integrating evidence-based solutions that support a foundation for EBP project implementation.
6. Integrate AACN *Essentials*.

12-WEEK SYLLABUS WITH SIX TWO-WEEK MODULES

Module 1 (Weeks 1–2): Conducting a Comprehensive Literature Review

Learning Objectives
- Conduct a comprehensive literature review using JHEBP and PRISMA frameworks (CLO1).
- Apply AACN *Essentials* IV (Scholarship for the DNP) and V (Information Systems/Technology) by utilizing advanced literature review methodologies.

Topics
- Overview of the JHEBP literature review tool and PRISMA framework
- Systematic search strategies and data extraction

Activities
- **Workshop:** Introduction to the JHEBP Evidence Summary Tools (Appendices G1 and G2) and PRISMA flow diagram for managing systematic reviews
- **Database Exercise:** Guided literature search using PubMed, CINAHL, and Cochrane Library

Assignments
- **Literature Search Report:** Submit a report detailing the search strategy, databases used, and preliminary results with a PRISMA flow diagram.
- **Discussion Post:** Reflect on challenges and successes encountered in conducting the literature search.

Module 2 (Weeks 3–4): Evidence Evaluation and Synthesis

Learning Objectives
- Evaluate and synthesize the body of evidence to identify evidence-based solutions for clinical issues (CLO2).
- Align with AACN *Essentials* IV (Scholarship for the DNP) and VIII (Clinical Scholarship) by conducting evidence appraisal to inform practice decisions.

Topics
- Critical appraisal of studies and synthesis of evidence
- Using JHEBP's Appendix H (Summary, Synthesis, & Best-Evidence Recommendations Tool) for grading the evidence

Activities
- Case Study Analysis: Apply Appendix H to sample studies for practice.
- Group Discussion: Analyze and discuss the quality and relevance of key evidence for the practice question.

Assignments
- Evidence Evaluation Matrix: Submit an evidence evaluation matrix summarizing key articles, their evidence levels, and applicability.
- Discussion Post: Present and discuss findings from one appraised study with peers.

Module 3 (Weeks 5–6): Refining Project AIMS With SMART Goals

Learning Objectives
- Refine project AIMS using the SMART format (CLO3).
- Integrate AACN *Essentials* II (Organizational Leadership) and VIII (Clinical Scholarship) by creating targeted, measurable project goals.

Topics
- Developing SMART goals (Specific, Measurable, Achievable, Relevant, Time-bound)
- Aligning AIMS with evidence-based findings and organizational priorities

Activities
- Workshop: Construct and refine project AIMS based on evidence synthesis.
- Peer Review: Share and receive feedback on AIMS statements with classmates.

Assignments
- SMART Goals Worksheet: Complete and submit a worksheet with refined AIMS for the project.
- Discussion Post: Share your SMART AIMS and discuss how the evidence informs each goal.

Module 4 (Weeks 7–8): Assessing Organizational Readiness for EBP Implementation

Learning Objectives
- Assess organizational readiness for implementing evidence-based changes (CLO4).
- Apply AACN *Essentials* II (Organizational Leadership) and VI (Interprofessional Collaboration) to assess readiness and foster impacted groups engagement.

Topics
- Using the Impacted Groups Analysis and Communication Resource (Hopkins.org/resources) and the Translation Tool (Appendix I)
- Strategies for effective impacted groups engagement and assessing readiness

Activities
- Simulation Exercise: Conduct a mock organizational readiness assessment using Appendix I and other resources.
- Impacted Groups Mapping: Use the Impacted Groups Analysis and Communication Resource to identify and map key impacted groups.

Assignments
- Readiness Assessment Report: Submit an organizational readiness assessment report summarizing findings from Appendix I.
- Impacted Groups Engagement Plan: Develop a plan outlining communication strategies for engaging impacted groups.

Module 5 (Weeks 9–10): Developing a Preliminary Project Plan

Learning Objectives
- Develop a preliminary project plan that integrates evidence-based solutions (CLO5).
- Incorporate AACN *Essentials* II (Organizational and Systems Leadership) and IX (Mastery of Advanced Nursing Practice) by creating a plan that considers organizational processes and systems.

Topics
- Outlining project activities and resource requirements
- Setting timelines and defining project milestones

Activities
- Workshop: Introduction to Appendix H and develop a project plan.
- Group Exercise: Draft a project plan outline and give and receive peer feedback.

Assignments
- Preliminary Project Plan: Submit an outline of the preliminary project plan, including key activities, timeline, and milestones.
- Discussion Post: Share key components of the project plan with peers and discuss potential challenges.

Module 6 (Weeks 11–12): Integrative Review Paper and Final Project Plan Submission

Learning Objectives
- Integrate evidence-based solutions into a cohesive project plan and prepare for implementation (CLO5).
- Emphasize AACN *Essentials* VIII (Clinical Scholarship) and IX (Mastery of Advanced Nursing Practice) by synthesizing evidence into a formal project plan.

Topics
- Writing an integrative review and refining the project plan
- Preparing the final project plan and next steps for implementation

Activities
- Peer Review: Exchange and review final project plans with classmates.
- Group Reflection: Discuss lessons learned and strategies for effective project translation.

Assignments
- Integrative Review Paper: Submit a 10–12-page integrative review paper including:
  - Project AIMS (SMART goals)
  - Organizational readiness assessment
  - Preliminary project plan
- Presentation: Deliver a five-to-seven-minute presentation on the project plan and integrative review to the class.
- Reflection Journal: Reflect on the experience of connecting evidence to project planning and readiness assessment.

Evaluation and Grading
- Discussion Participation – 15%
- Literature Search Report (Module 1) – 10%
- Evidence Evaluation Matrix (Module 2) – 10%
- SMART Goals Worksheet (Module 3) – 10%
- Readiness Assessment Report and Impacted Groups Engagement Plan (Module 4) – 15%
- Preliminary Project Plan (Module 5) – 10%
- Integrative Review Paper and Presentation (Module 6) – 30%

PROJECT COURSE #3: CONNECTING THE EVIDENCE FOR PROJECT TRANSLATION

Practice Question → Evidence → Translation

Course Objectives
- Engage in collaborative discussions with organizational representatives to present literature review findings and assess the feasibility of identified evidence-based solutions within the clinical setting.
- Analyze and apply the science of translation using the JHEBP model, selecting an appropriate translational framework that aligns with project goals and organizational needs.
- Evaluate the fit and feasibility of proposed interventions by critically assessing organizational readiness, refining implementation strategies, and developing a finalized action plan for translating evidence into practice.
- AACN *Essentials* Level 2 Professional Nursing Education sub-competencies and domains (AACN, 2021, pp. 17–58)
- Melnyk & Fineout-Overholt EBP Competencies in Graduate Programs: #14–16, 17–19, & 23

Course Activities/Assignments
- Learners engage with project site impacted groups, leaders, and clinical experts specific to the project topic, population, and preliminary EBP intervention (QI) or proposal.
- Practicum hours: 56 hours
- Learners critically appraise, synthesize the literature, and integrate the findings to develop an EBP project action plan for a healthcare intervention or a process improvement ("translating evidence to construct a strategy or method to address a problem and designing a plan for implementation and actual implementation when possible" [AACN, 2021, p. 24]).
- Learners formulate project SMART goals or aims reflecting the problem statement, PICO question, and/or purpose statement for the project action plan and consider the impact of patient care/provider practice on either a direct QI/(live) or indirection project (exploratory/PI).
- Learners develop a Work Breakdown Structure (WBS) plan and/or a Gantt chart to reflect the project timeline and identify the strengths, weaknesses, opportunities, and threats of the project (SWOT) and risk mitigation strategies.

- Learners identify the data collection and methodology plan to evaluate data outcomes measurements (QI or PI), such as the tools or surveys or aggregate data/rates collection to present the results, assess feasibility and sustainability, and/or expert critique and review for future QI.
- Learners utilize and continue to refine:
  - Gantt chart
  - Translation Tool (see Appendix I)
  - Impacted Groups Analysis and Communication Resource (Hopkins.org/resources)
  - Formulate an Implementation and Action Planning (A-3) Tool (Appendix J)
- Learners will present the developed action plan to the appropriate approval unit (agency or university IRB, etc.) for review to translate the project's action plan.

SAMPLE DNP PROJECT COURSE #3 SYLLABUS

EXPLORING THE EVIDENCE, TRANSLATIONAL FRAMEWORKS, AND INITIAL ACTION PLANNING

Course Description

In this course, students will collaborate closely with organizational representatives to present findings from their literature review and assess the feasibility of identified evidence-based solutions. Students will explore the science of translation within the JHEBP model, focusing on selecting an appropriate translational framework that aligns with their project goals and organizational needs. This course guides students in assessing the fit and feasibility of their proposed interventions, fostering critical thinking to determine the best approach for evidence translation. By the end of the course, students will choose a translational framework and finalize an action plan to implement their proposed solutions within the organization.

Key JHEBP Tools: Appendix B, Appendix I, Appendix C

Competency-Based Assessment: Selection of a translational framework and a finalized action plan in collaboration with the organizational mentor

Course Learning Objectives (CLOs)

1. Present literature review findings to organizational representatives.
2. Explore the science of translation and assess different translational frameworks.
3. Assess the fit and feasibility of proposed interventions within the organizational context.
4. Finalize the action plan in collaboration with the organizational mentor, preparing for implementation.
5. Integrate AACN *Essentials*.

12-WEEK SYLLABUS WITH SIX TWO-WEEK MODULES

Module 1 (Weeks 1–2): Presenting Literature Review Findings and Gathering Organizational Feedback

Learning Objectives
- Present literature review findings to organizational representatives (CLO1).
- Gather feedback on the feasibility of evidence-based solutions within the organization.
- Integrate AACN *Essentials* VI (Interprofessional Collaboration) and VIII (Clinical Scholarship) by sharing findings and gathering feedback from organizational representatives.

Topics
- Strategies for effectively communicating evidence-based findings to impacted groups
- Collecting feedback and understanding organizational constraints

Activities
- Workshop: Learn presentation skills and prepare evidence-based findings for impacted groups.
- Feedback Session: Present literature review findings to a small group, simulating organizational feedback sessions.

Assignments
- Literature Review Presentation: Prepare and deliver a presentation of literature review findings to organizational representatives (real or simulated).
- Discussion Post: Reflect on feedback received and discuss implications for the proposed intervention.

Module 2 (Weeks 3–4): Introduction to Translational Science and Frameworks

Learning Objectives
- Explore the science of translation and assess different translational frameworks (CLO2).
- Apply AACN *Essentials* IV (Scholarship for the DNP) and IX (Mastery of Advanced Nursing Practice) by evaluating translational frameworks for project use.

Topics
- Overview of translational science and EBP models
- Introduction to various translational frameworks (e.g., Knowledge-to-Action, RE-AIM, PARIHS)

Activities
- Case Study Review: Analyze examples of translational frameworks applied in clinical settings.
- Group Discussion: Compare different frameworks and discuss their strengths and weaknesses.

Assignments
- Translational Framework Comparison: Write a short paper comparing at least two translational frameworks and discussing their potential fit with your project.
- Discussion Post: Share insights on the frameworks considered and initial thoughts on which might best align with the project.

Module 3 (Weeks 5–6): Selecting a Translational Framework for the Project

Learning Objectives
- Select an appropriate translational framework that aligns with project goals and organizational needs (CLO2).
- Integrate AACN *Essential* IX (Mastery of Advanced Nursing Practice) by selecting a framework to guide evidence translation.

Topics
- Applying the JHEBP model to guide framework selection
- Considering organizational culture, mission, and resources in framework selection

Activities
- Workshop: Using Appendix B (Question Development Tool) to refine the practice question and ensure alignment with the chosen framework.
- Peer Review Session: Share framework choices with peers and receive feedback on fit and feasibility.

Assignments
- Framework Selection Justification: Submit a two-to-three-page paper justifying the choice of translational framework and how it aligns with the project and organizational context.
- Discussion Post: Discuss the rationale for the selected framework and anticipated challenges.

Module 4 (Weeks 7–8): Assessing Fit and Feasibility of Proposed Interventions

Learning Objectives

- Assess the fit and feasibility of proposed interventions within the organizational context (CLO3).
- Apply AACN *Essential* II (Organizational and Systems Leadership) and VI (Interprofessional Collaboration) by ensuring proposed interventions align with organizational needs and resources.

Topics

- Evaluating resources, organizational readiness, and impacted groups perspectives
- Using the Translation Tool (Appendix I) for readiness assessment

Activities

- Simulation Exercise: Conduct a mock readiness assessment with Appendix I.
- Impacted Groups Mapping Exercise: Identify impacted groups and their roles in the project implementation.

Assignments

- Feasibility Assessment Report: Submit a report that summarizes the feasibility assessment findings, including resources, potential barriers, and facilitators.
- Discussion Post: Share findings on feasibility and discuss any adjustments needed to improve alignment with the organization.

Module 5 (Weeks 9–10): Developing an Initial Action Plan

Learning Objectives

- Begin developing a finalized action plan for implementing proposed solutions (CLO4).
- Align with AACN *Essential* II (Organizational and Systems Leadership) by creating an actionable plan that considers organizational processes and systems.

Topics

- Creating actionable steps, timelines, and setting short- and long-term goals
- Integrating impacted groups feedback into the action plan

Activities

- Workshop: Outline the key components of an effective action plan and align project goals with organizational timelines.
- Group Exercise: Draft a preliminary action plan and give and receive peer feedback.

Assignments

- Preliminary Action Plan: Submit a draft of the action plan, including key activities, resource needs, and a timeline.
- Discussion Post: Present the preliminary plan and discuss feedback from organizational impacted groups.

Module 6 (Weeks 11–12): Finalizing the Action Plan and Preparing for Implementation

Learning Objectives

- Finalize the action plan in collaboration with the organizational mentor, preparing for implementation (CLO4).
- Embrace AACN *Essential* IX (Mastery of Advanced Nursing Practice) by demonstrating advanced skills in action planning and preparation for implementation.

Topics

- Refining the action plan based on final feedback and aligning with the chosen translational framework
- Preparing for the next course and implementation phase

Activities

- Mentor Review Session: Review the final action plan with the organizational mentor to ensure alignment with organizational goals.
- Reflection Activity: Reflect on the process of selecting a framework, assessing feasibility, and preparing the action plan.

Assignments

- Final Action Plan: Submit a comprehensive action plan (10–12 pages) that includes:
  - Literature review summary
  - Selected translational framework and justification
  - Feasibility assessment results
  - Finalized action steps, timeline, and resource needs
- Presentation: Deliver a brief presentation summarizing the action plan and its alignment with organizational goals.
- Reflection Journal: Reflect on the challenges and learning experiences in preparing for the project's implementation phase.

Evaluation and Grading

- Discussion Participation – 15%
- Literature Review Presentation (Module 1) – 10%
- Translational Framework Comparison (Module 2) – 10%
- Framework Selection Justification (Module 3) – 10%
- Feasibility Assessment Report (Module 4) – 15%
- Preliminary Action Plan (Module 5) – 10%
- Final Action Plan and Presentation (Module 6) – 30%

PROJECT COURSE #4: TRANSLATION OF PROJECT ACTION PLAN

Practice Question → Evidence → Translation

Course Objectives

- Develop and apply data collection, analysis, and interpretation skills to generate evidence that informs and improves nursing practice, aligning with the DNP *Essentials* and EBP principles.

- Integrate advanced nursing practice scholarship with organizational leadership by utilizing data-driven methodologies for quality improvement and evidence translation, ensuring alignment with healthcare systems and organizational priorities.

- Demonstrate scholarly dissemination of project outcomes through the creation of formal written reports and presentations, effectively communicating research findings to influence practice change and improve patient outcomes.

- AACN *Essentials* Level 2 Professional Nursing Education sub-competencies and domains (AACN, 2021, pp. 17–58)

- Melnyk & Fineout-Overholt EBP Competencies in Graduate Programs: #14–16, 17–19, & 23

Course Activities/Assignments

- Learners engage with project site impacted groups, leaders, and clinical experts specific to the project topic, population, and preliminary EBP intervention (QI) or proposal for active project translation.

- Practicum hours: 56 hours

- Gantt chart: continue work on

- Learners will launch/implement the developed action plan (aims) and begin data collection methods; translation leaders will translate either the direct or indirect project action plan and evaluate the impact of patient care/provider practice:

    1. QI/Traditional DNP Project: Live implementation of aims interventions:

        - Data methods/gathering align with QI: pre/post intervention design or aggregate data collection (chart review or tool usage, etc.)

2. Exploratory Project/PI:
   - Implementation of action plan of project aims and measure project outcomes (QI)
   - Query experts on feasibility and sustainability (PI)
   - Learners can develop and distribute a virtual module/bundle of a proposal using various resources:
     - AHRQ bundle sets, proposed tools/flowcharts, educational inservice modules, assistance with grant proposal/submission/NGOs, legislative activity, etc.
     - Bundle for Magnet® qualifications or continual certification.
   - Translate the data analysis and methods: Appraise and assess pre/post tools, surveys, and/or critiques from expert clinicians/team members on the developed action plan (the material, bundle, tool, grant application, policy, etc.)
   - Begin to assess and critically integrate post-critique feedback and analyze what changes are needed for improvement (see Figure 5.3) and revise accordingly

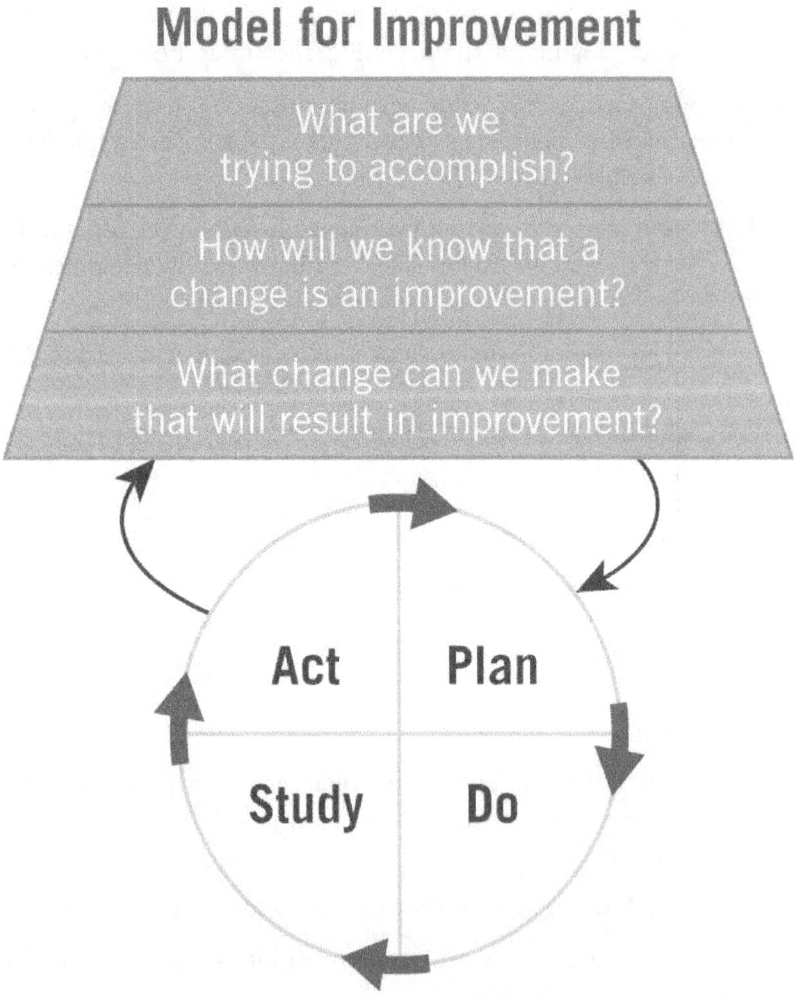

Model for Improvement

- What are we trying to accomplish?
- How will we know that a change is an improvement?
- What change can we make that will result in improvement?

Act — Plan
Study — Do

FIGURE 5.3 Model for improvement.

SAMPLE DNP PROJECT COURSE #4 SYLLABUS

TRANSLATION OF PROJECT ACTION PLAN

Course Description
This course provides DNP students with the skills to collect, analyze, and interpret data to generate evidence that informs nursing practice. Students will develop databases, analyze data to predict or evaluate improvements, and summarize results in scholarly formats. For DNP/AP and DNP executive students in practicum, this course integrates advanced nursing practice scholarship with organizational leadership, quality improvement, and evidence translation. The course aligns with the AACN *Essentials* and emphasizes the scholarly dissemination of project outcomes through formal written reports and presentations.

Course Learning Objectives (CLOs)
Upon successful completion of this course, students will be able to:

1. Collect appropriate data to generate evidence for nursing practice.

2. Develop databases and/or information sets that generate meaningful evidence for practice.

3. Analyze data/information to inform, predict, and/or evaluate practice or practice improvements.

4. Summarize project results in a scholarly written report consistent with JHSON evaluation criteria for the DNP scholarly project report.

5. Disseminate the results of the DNP project through a formal presentation consistent with JHSON evaluation criteria for the DNP scholarly project presentation.

6. For DNP/AP and DNP executive students in practicum, integrate principles of advanced nursing practice scholarship to improve outcomes through organizational/system leadership, quality improvement processes, and translation of evidence into practice to meet the AACN *Essentials*.

EIGHT-WEEK SYLLABUS

Week 1: Introduction to Data Collection in Nursing Practice
- Understanding the importance of data in evidence-based nursing practice
- Activity: Identifying data sources and collection methods
- Assignment: Develop a data collection plan for your project (CLO1)

Week 2: Building Databases and Information Sets
- Developing and organizing databases to store project data
- Activity: Database creation and management exercise
- Assignment: Design a database or information set for your project (CLO2)

Week 3: Data Analysis for Practice Improvement
- Statistical and qualitative data analysis techniques
- Activity: Data analysis practice using real-world data sets
- Assignment: Analyze a sample data set and interpret the results (CLO3)

Week 4: Scholarly Writing for DNP Projects
- Structuring a scholarly report based on data findings
- Activity: Reviewing JHSON scholarly project report guidelines
- Assignment: Submit a draft of your scholarly report based on project data (CLO4)

Week 5: Presentation Skills and Dissemination of Results
- Techniques for presenting research findings to diverse audiences
- Activity: Developing visual aids for presentations (e.g., slides, charts)
- Assignment: Create a presentation outline for your project (CLO5)

Week 6: Organizational Leadership and Quality Improvement
- Integrating data analysis with leadership in quality improvement
- Activity: Case study on leading quality improvement initiatives
- Assignment: Proposal for a quality improvement process informed by data analysis (CLO6)

Week 7: Translating Evidence into Practice
- Applying evidence generated from data analysis to improve practice
- Activity: Translating project findings into actionable practice recommendations
- Assignment: Finalize and submit a plan for evidence translation in a clinical setting (CLO6)

Week 8: Final Project Presentation and Report Submission
- Presenting project findings and submitting the final report
- Activity: Project presentations and peer evaluations
- Assignment: Final project presentation and written report (CLO4–CLO5)

Evaluation and Grading
- Data Collection Plan (CLO1): 15%
- Database/Information Set Design (CLO2): 15%
- Data Analysis Assignment (CLO3): 20%
- Draft Scholarly Report (CLO4): 15%
- Presentation Outline (CLO5): 15%
- Quality Improvement Proposal (CLO6): 20%

PROJECT COURSE #5: EVALUATION OF THE TRANSLATION AND DISSEMINATION

Practice Question → Evidence → Translation

Course Objectives
- Evaluate the impact of an evidence-based intervention by analyzing project data, measuring outcomes, and assessing sustainability within the organization to determine its effectiveness in improving clinical practice and healthcare outcomes.
- Develop a comprehensive dissemination plan to share project findings with key stakeholders, professional organizations, and academic audiences through presentations, conference submissions, or scholarly publications.
- Synthesize project outcomes into a scholarly paper, integrating data evaluation, interpretation, and dissemination strategies to contribute to EBP and future healthcare improvements.
- AACN *Essentials* Level 2 Professional Nursing Education sub-competencies and domains (AACN, 2021, pp. 17–58)
- Melnyk & Fineout-Overholt EBP Competencies in Graduate Programs: # 14–16, 17–19, 20, 21, 23, & 24
- Demonstrate competencies in all 24 EBP Integration Competencies.

Course Activities/Assignments: In Collaboration With 808 Data Analyses Course
- Learners engage with project site impacted groups, leaders, and clinical experts specific to the project topic, population, and preliminary EBP intervention (QI) or proposal for evaluation and dissemination.
- Practicum hours: 56 hours
- Learners will conduct an "evaluation of the outcomes, process, and/or experience" of the action plan experience/work (AACN, 2021, p. 24).
- Translation evaluation: Learners will discover and evaluate either the direct or indirect project action plan and analyze the impact of patient care/provider practice.
- Gantt chart: continue work on

- Examine and evaluate the evidence of the data through analysis and evaluation methods: Appraise and assess pre/post tools, surveys, and/or critiques from expert clinicians/team members on the developed action plan—the material, bundle, tool, grant application, policy, etc.—the measures used that align with the action project's aims or goals and aligns with the project's purpose/problem statement and/or PICO question.

- Systematically assess and critically integrate post critique feedback and analyze what changes are needed for improvement and revise accordingly.

- Dissemination and presentation to impacted groups:
    1. Poster and/or PowerPoint presentation to impacted groups and/or agency leaders
    2. Explore, describe, and disseminate the project's results and outcomes on patient care outcomes: Will the project become the site's best practices or is more revision needed? (PDSA cycle)
        a. If QI: Will the EBP best practice intervention become standard practice and/or be incorporated into the project site's patient care or provider practice/education? (feasibility and sustainability)
        b. If a PI: Further query, revisions, and/or actions needed to secure a future QI project?

- Learners: Final paper or manuscript as per appropriate journal (student can choose)
- Appendix J

SAMPLE DNP PROJECT COURSE #5 SYLLABUS

PROJECT EVALUATION AND DISSEMINATION

Course Description

This final course guides students through the evaluation of their evidence-based project, focusing on outcome measurement and sustainability within the organization. Students will analyze project data to determine the impact of their intervention on clinical practice and healthcare outcomes. Additionally, the course emphasizes the importance of dissemination, providing students with strategies to share their findings with impacted groups, professional conferences, or academic publications. By the end of this course, students will have a complete evaluation of their project and a clear plan for sharing their work to drive future evidence-based improvements in healthcare. The students will also write their scholarly paper to include their data evaluation and dissemination plan.

Key JHEBP Tools: Appendix I, DNP Scholarly PPT, other appendices as needed

Competency-Based Assessment: Completed project evaluation report and dissemination plan

Course Learning Objectives (CLOs)

1. Evaluate the outcomes of the evidence-based project by analyzing project data to assess the impact on clinical practice and healthcare outcomes.

2. Develop strategies for sustaining project results within the organization to ensure long-term improvements.

3. Create a dissemination plan to effectively share project findings with key impacted groups, professional audiences, and academic communities.

4. Prepare a comprehensive scholarly paper that includes data evaluation, sustainability recommendations, and dissemination strategies to drive future evidence-based improvements.

5. Integrate AACN *Essentials*.

12-WEEK SYLLABUS WITH SIX TWO-WEEK MODULES

Module 1 (Weeks 1–2): Analyzing Project Outcomes and Data Evaluation

Learning Objectives
- Evaluate the outcomes of the evidence-based project using data analysis techniques (CLO1).
- Integrate AACN *Essentials* IV (Scholarship for the DNP) and V (Information Systems/Technology) by applying analytical methods to assess the effectiveness of clinical interventions.

Topics
- Techniques for analyzing quantitative and qualitative data
- Assessing the impact of interventions on clinical and organizational outcomes

Activities
- Workshop: Review data analysis methods for healthcare outcomes.
- Group Exercise: Practice interpreting data with sample project results.

Assignments
- Data Analysis Report: Submit an initial report analyzing your project data, including descriptive statistics, trends, and key findings.
- Discussion Post: Share preliminary analysis insights and challenges with peers.

Module 2 (Weeks 3–4): Interpreting Results and Assessing Impact

Learning Objectives
- Interpret project results to understand the clinical and organizational impact of the intervention (CLO1).
- Apply AACN *Essential* IX (Mastery of Advanced Nursing Practice) by using data interpretation to guide future practice and organizational decisions.

Topics
- Interpreting data in the context of EBP
- Identifying key findings and implications for clinical practice and organizational outcomes

Activities
- Case Study Analysis: Examine case studies of successful project evaluations and discuss interpretation approaches.
- Peer Review Session: Share and receive feedback on data interpretation.

Assignments
- Impact Assessment Report: Submit a report summarizing the implications of your findings for clinical and organizational practice.
- Discussion Post: Discuss the real-world impact of your project and explore how the findings can inform future practice.

Module 3 (Weeks 5–6): Planning for Project Sustainability

Learning Objectives
- Develop strategies for sustaining the positive impact of the project within the organization (CLO2).
- Integrate AACN *Essential* II (Organizational and Systems Leadership) by creating sustainability plans to support long-term improvements in healthcare outcomes.

Topics
- Strategies for maintaining change, including resource allocation and impacted groups engagement
- Identifying barriers and facilitators to project sustainability

Activities
- Workshop: Practice strategies for promoting project sustainability in clinical and organizational settings.
- Group Discussion: Share ideas for overcoming potential barriers to long-term success.

Assignments
- Sustainability Plan: Develop a detailed sustainability plan outlining steps, resources, and impacted groups involvement.
- Discussion Post: Discuss the sustainability plan and strategies for ensuring ongoing project impact.

Module 4 (Weeks 7–8): Developing a Dissemination Plan

Learning Objectives

- Create a dissemination plan to share project findings with impacted groups, professional conferences, and academic audiences (CLO3).
- Align with AACN *Essential* VII (Clinical Prevention and Population Health) by targeting dissemination strategies that contribute to improved population health outcomes.

Topics

- Identifying appropriate dissemination channels (e.g., presentations, publications, internal reports)
- Preparing for conference presentations, poster sessions, and academic publication

Activities

- Workshop: Crafting an effective dissemination plan and targeting specific audiences.
- Peer Review: Share dissemination ideas with classmates and receive feedback on potential channels and strategies.

Assignments

- Dissemination Plan Submission: Develop and submit a plan detailing specific audiences, channels, and timelines for dissemination.
- Discussion Post: Discuss the chosen dissemination strategies and the impact on advancing evidence-based practices.

Module 5 (Weeks 9–10): Writing the Scholarly Paper

Learning Objectives

- Prepare a scholarly paper that integrates data evaluation, sustainability, and dissemination strategies (CLO4).
- Fulfill AACN *Essential* VIII (Advanced Practice) by writing a scholarly paper that showcases project evaluation and mastery in evidence-based improvements.

Topics

- Structuring the scholarly paper to include project background, data analysis, findings, sustainability, and dissemination
- Writing for publication and professional audiences

Activities
- Writing Workshop: Guidance on organizing and drafting sections of the scholarly paper.
- Peer Feedback: Exchange drafts of key sections and provide constructive feedback.

Assignments
- Scholarly Paper Draft Submission: Submit a draft of the scholarly paper, covering project outcomes, sustainability, and dissemination strategies.
- Discussion Post: Reflect on the writing process and challenges in presenting data and findings effectively.

Module 6 (Weeks 11–12): Finalizing and Presenting the Scholarly Project

Learning Objectives
- Finalize the scholarly paper and deliver a presentation on the project's impact, sustainability, and dissemination (CLO4).
- Embrace AACN *Essential* VI (Interprofessional Collaboration) by presenting project findings to diverse audiences and highlighting collaborative impacts on healthcare improvement.

Topics
- Presenting data and outcomes effectively to diverse audiences
- Reflection on project outcomes and impact on personal and professional development

Activities
- Final Presentation: Prepare and deliver a presentation on the scholarly project, summarizing data analysis, sustainability, and dissemination plans.
- Reflection Activity: Reflect on the journey from project initiation to dissemination and future directions.

Assignments
- Final Scholarly Paper Submission: Submit the final version of the scholarly paper, including all required components.
- Presentation to Class or Impacted Groups: Present the project findings, impact, and future directions to peers and faculty.
- Reflection Journal: Write a final reflection on the project process, learning outcomes, and professional growth.

Evaluation and Grading
- Discussion Participation – 15%
- Data Analysis Report (Module 1) – 10%
- Impact Assessment Report (Module 2) – 10%
- Sustainability Plan (Module 3) – 10%
- Dissemination Plan Submission (Module 4) – 15%
- Scholarly Paper Draft (Module 5) – 10%
- Final Scholarly Paper and Presentation (Module 6) – 30%

REFERENCES

Al Zoubi, F., Mayo, N., Rochette, A., & Thomas, A. (2018). Applying modern measurement approaches to constructs relevant to evidence-based practice among Canadian physical and occupational therapists. *Implementation Science, 13*(1), 152. https://doi.org/10.1186/s13012-018-0844-4

American Association of Colleges of Nursing. (2008). *The essentials of baccalaureate education for professional nursing practice.* https://www.aacnnursing.org/Portals/42/Publications/BaccEssentials08.pdf

American Association of Colleges of Nursing. (2011). *The essentials of master's education in nursing.* www.aacnnursing.org/Portals/42/Publications/MastersEssentials11.pdf

American Association of Colleges of Nursing. (2021). *The essentials: Core competencies for professional nursing education.* https://www.aacnnursing.org/Portals/0/PDFs/Publications/Essentials-2021.pdf

Bissett, K., Ascenzi, J., & Whalen, M. (2025). *Johns Hopkins evidence-based practice for nurses and healthcare professionals: Model & guidelines* (5th ed.). Sigma Theta Tau International.

Centers for Disease Control and Prevention. (2018, August). *Data collection methods for program evaluation: Focus groups.* https://www.cdc.gov/healthy-youth/php/program-evaluation/pdf/brief17.pdf

Dang, D., Dearholt, S. L., Bissett, K., Ascenzi, J., & Whalen, M. (2021). *Johns Hopkins evidence-based practice for nurses and healthcare professionals: Model & guidelines* (4th ed.). Sigma Theta Tau International.

English, F. W., & Kaufman, R. A. (1975). *Needs assessment: A focus for curriculum development.* Association for Supervision and Curriculum Development.

Fernandez-Dominguez, J. C., Sese-Abad, A., Morales-Asencio, J. M., Sastre-Fullana, P., Pol-Castaneda, S., & de Pedro-Gomez, J. E. (2016). Content validity of a health science evidence-based practice questionnaire (HS-EBP) with a web-based modified Delphi approach. *International Journal for Quality in Health Care, 28*(6), 764–773. https://doi.org/10.1093/intqhc/mzw106

Institute for Healthcare Improvement. (n.d.). *Model for improvement: Forming the team.* https://www.ihi.org/how-improve-model-improvement-forming-team

Kaper, N. M., Swennen, M. H., van Wijk, A. J., Kalkman, C. J., van Rheenen, N., van der Graaf, Y., & van der Heijden, G. J. M. G. (2015). The "evidence-based practice inventory": Reliability and validity was demonstrated for a novel instrument to identify barriers and facilitators for evidence-based practice in health care. *Journal of Clinical Epidemiology, 68*(11), 1261–1269. https://doi.org/10.1016/j.jclinepi.2015.06.002

Karlsen, J. T. (2020). The project steering committee, project governance and trust: Insights from a practical case study. *Management Research Review, 44*(6), 926–947. https://doi.org/10.1108/MRR-12-2019-0540

Landsverk, N. G., Olsen, N. R., & Brovold, T. (2023, Sept. 13). Instruments measuring evidence-based practice behavior, attitudes, and self-efficacy among healthcare professionals: A systematic review of measurement properties. *Implementation Science, 18*(1), 42. https://doi.org/10.1186/s13012-023-01301-3

Lim, B. C., & Klein, K. J. (2006). Team mental models and team performance: A field study of the effects of team mental model similarity and accuracy. *Journal of Organizational Behavior, 27*(4), 403–418. https://psycnet.apa.org/doi/10.1002/job.387

Marczak, M., & Sewell, M. (n.d.). *Using focus groups for evaluation.* University of Arizona. https://cales.arizona.edu/sfcs/cyfernet/cyfar/focus.htm

McEvoy, M. P., Williams, M. T., & Olds, T. S. (2010). Development and psychometric testing of a trans-professional evidence-based practice profile questionnaire. *Medical Teacher, 32*(9), e373–e380. https://doi.org/10.3109/0142159x.2010.494741

Melnyk, B. M., & Fineout-Overholt, E. (2019). *Evidence-based practice in nursing & healthcare* (4th ed.). Wolters Kluwer.

Melnyk, B. M., & Fineout-Overholt, E. (2023). *Evidence-based practice in nursing & healthcare* (5th ed.). Wolters Kluwer.

Migliore, L., Chouinard, H., & Woodlee, R. (2020). Clinical research and practice collaborative: An evidence-based nursing clinical inquiry expansion. *Military Medicine, 185*(Suppl. 2), 35–42. https://doi.org/10.1093/milmed/usz447

Moran, K., Burson, R., & Conrad, D. (2024). *The doctor of nursing practice scholarly project: A framework for success* (4th ed.). Jones & Bartlett Learning.

Mueller, J. S. (2012). Why individuals in larger teams perform worse. *Organizational Behavior & Human Decision Processes, 117*(1), 111–124. https://doi.org/10.1016/j.obhdp.2011.08.004

Newhouse, R. P., & Spring, B. (2010, November–December). Interdisciplinary evidence-based practice: Moving from silos to synergy. *Nursing Outlook, 58*(6), 309–317. https://doi.org/10.1016/j.outlook.2010.09.001

Onwuegbuzie, A. J., Dickinson, W. B., Leech, N. L., & Zoran, A. G. (2009). A qualitative framework for collecting and analyzing data in focus group research. *International Journal of Qualitative Methods, 8*(3), 1–21. https://doi.org/10.1177/160940690900800301

OpenAI. (2024). *ChatGPT* (version 4o) [Large language model]. https://chatgpt.com

Ruano, A. S. M., Motter, F. R., & Lopes, L. C. (2022, April 8). Design and validity of an instrument to assess healthcare professionals' perceptions, behaviour, self-efficacy and attitudes towards evidence-based health practice: I-SABE. *BMJ Open, 12*(4), e052767. https://doi.org/10.1136/bmjopen-2021-052767

Rubin, A., & Parrish, D. E. (2010). Development and validation of the Evidence-based Practice Process Assessment Scale: Preliminary findings. *Research on Social Work Practice, 20*(6), 629–640. https://doi.org/10.1177/1049731508329420

University of Mississippi. (2005). *Guidelines for conducting a focus group.* Eliot & Associates. https://irep.olemiss.edu/wpcontent/uploads/sites/98/2016/05/Trinity_Duke_How_to_Conduct_a_Focus_Group.pdf

Verzuh, E. (2021). *Fast forward MBA in project management* (6th ed.). Wiley.

www.ingramcontent.com/pod-product-compliance
Lightning Source LLC
Chambersburg PA
CBHW082209300426
44117CB00016B/2727